John Cooke, John Maule

An historical account of the Royal Hospital for Seamen at Greenwich

M,DCC,LXXXIX

John Cooke, John Maule

An historical account of the Royal Hospital for Seamen at Greenwich
M,DCC,LXXXIX

ISBN/EAN: 9783741185359

Manufactured in Europe, USA, Canada, Australia, Japa

Cover: Foto ©Andreas Hilbeck / pixelio.de

Manufactured and distributed by brebook publishing software
(www.brebook.com)

John Cooke, John Maule

An historical account of the Royal Hospital for Seamen at Greenwich

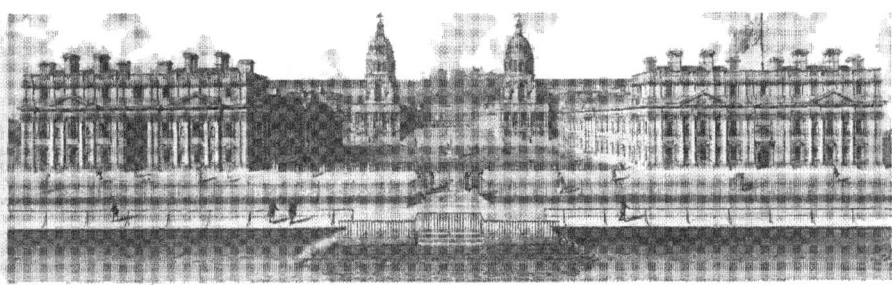

A perspective View of the Royal Hospital for Seamen at Greenwich taken from the River Thames

A N

HISTORICAL ACCOUNT

OF THE

ROYAL HOSPITAL

FOR

SEAMEN

AT

GREENWICH.

M,DCC,LXXXIX.

Garrula fecuri narrare pericula Nautæ.

Juv. Sat.

LONDON:

SOLD FOR THE AUTHORS BY

G. NICOL, PALL-MALL; T. CADELL, STRAND; J. WALTER, CHARING-CROSS;
G. G. J. AND J. ROBINSON, PATER-NOSTER-ROW;

AND

AT THE CHAPEL OF THE HOSPITAL.

Entered at Stationers-Hall.

TO THE

RIGHT HONORABLE THE LORDS AND OTHERS

COMMISSIONERS AND GOVERNORS

OF THE

ROYAL HOSPITAL FOR SEAMEN AT GREENWICH,

THE FOLLOWING HISTORICAL ACCOUNT,

COLLECTED BY PERMISSION,

FROM ORIGINAL PAPERS AND RECORDS,

AND EMBELLISHED WITH ENGRAVINGS,

I S,

WITH THE GREATEST RESPECT

AND DEFERENCE,

INSCRIBED, BY

THE AUTHORS,

JOHN COOKE, A.M. ⎱
JOHN MAULE, A.M. ⎰ Chaplains.

Royal Hospital for Seamen at Greenwich,
September 22d, 1789.

CONTENTS.

INTRO-

INTRODUCTION.

THERE is nothing which reflects greater honor upon human nature, than thofe Inftitutions which owe their rife to motives of Benevolence, and of fuch there are many and excellent in their kinds, the glory and ornament of thefe Kingdoms. But where we find attention to the relief of private diftrefs, joined to the moft effectual care of the public interefts, we cannot help admiring the political wifdom of fuch an Inftitution, whilft we are delighted with the reflection that it is the fource of happinefs to individuals. Inftitutions of this fort, however, requiring ability proportionable to the beneficial effects which they are meant to produce, cannot be fupported unlefs cherifhed by the ftreams of public Munificence, and the invigorating rays of Royal Favor.

With regard to that which it is our purpofe to trace from its Origin to its prefent ftate of Splendor,

dor, every one who wifhes well to this Country
muft with pleafure remark, how much its Interefts have been thought worthy the attention of
our Sovereigns, from the glorious Founders of it,
to the Prince who now fits upon the Throne,
whofe peculiar happinefs it is to promote and
encourage every undertaking which tends to the
Good of his People.

The Charaćter of piety and humanity which (a)
Hiftory has given to the Confort of William the
Third, appears to have been juftly founded;
many effects of her excellent difpofition remaining to this day. The firft idea of that noble
Inftitution, of which we are now treating, is
with every appearance of juftice afcribed to (b)
her. It was impoffible to find Objećts who
deferved better of the Public, or in a fituation
more deplorable, than thofe whofe Strength had
been exhaufted, or who had been mutilated or

(a) See her charaćter as drawn by Mr. Boyer in his Hiftory of King
William and Queen Mary.
(b) " And the laft great Projećt that her Thoughts were working
" upon, with relation to a noble and royal Provifion for difabled Seamen at
" Greenwich, was particularly defigned to be fo conftituted as to put them in a
" probable way of ending their Days in the Fear of God. "—See Boyer's above-
" mentioned Hiftory.

difabled

difabled in the fervice of their Country. For
want of a fafe harbour wherein they might
anchor, and an Afylum wherein they might
repofe, after the fatigues, hardfhips and dangers
which they had encountered, few only efcaped
from the accumulated diftreffes of poverty,
infirmity, and pain. To behold the Protectors
of a Nation which fhe loved, cruelly abandoned,
under fuch circumftances, excited her Royal
Compaffion; and one of the laft acts of her
exemplary Life was the propofal of an Inftitution,
which fhould provide for thofe unfortunate, but
highly deferving, Sufferers.

King William, fenfible of its utility, readily
acceded to the wifhes of his Royal Confort.
Before her demife, the following Grant was made
of a Houfe built by King Charles the Second,
with certain Lands in the Manor of Eaft Greenwich; and it will appear that, after the irreparable
Lofs which the Country and the King fuftained
by the Queen's deceafe, this Inftitution was
honored by his Majefty's fingular Protection.

Copy

Copy of King William's *and* Queen Mary's *Original Grant of* King Charles the Second's Palace *at* East-Greenwich, *and of the Ground thereto belonging, for the Use of an Hospital, for the Relief of Seamen, their Widows and Children.*

WILLIAM and MARY, by the Grace of God King & Queene of England, Scotland, France & Ireland, Defenders of the Faith, &c. to all to whome these Presents shall come Greeting. Whereas it is our Royal Intent and Recital of Intention to found an Hospital for Seamen. purpose to erect and found an Hospital within our Mannor of East Greenwich in our County of Kent for the reliefe and support of Seamen serving on board the Shipps or Vessells belonging to the Navy Royall of Us our Heires or Successors or imploy'd in our or their Service at Sea who by reason of Age Wounds or other disabilities shall be uncapable of further Service at Sea and be unable to maintain themselves And And for Sustentation of Widows, Children, and Relief of Seamen, &c. for the Sustentation of the Widows and the Maintenance and Education of the Children of Seamen happening to be slaine or disabled in such Sea Service and Also for the further reliefe and Encouragement of Seamen and Improvement of Navigation. Now to the End our Royal Purpose and Intention in the Premises may the better take Effect Know yee that Wee of our especial Grace certain Knowledge and

meere

meere Motion have givin and granted, and by thefe Prefents,
for us Our Heires and Succeffours doe give and grant unto
our right trufty and right well-beloved Counfellor S' John

Grant to certain Commiffioners Somers Kn' Keeper of our great Seale of England, our right
trufty and right entirely beloved Coufin & Counfellor Tho-
mas Duke of Leeds Prefident of our Privy Council our right
trufty and right well-beloved Coufin & Counfellor Tho'
Earle of Pembrooke and Montgomery Keeper of our Privy
Seale, our right trufty & right entirely beloved Coufin &
Counfellor Charles Duke of Shrewfbury one of our Principall Secretaries of State, our right trufty and well-beloved
Counfellor Sidney Lord Godolphin firft Commiffioner of
our Treafury, & our right trufty and well-beloved Counfellors S' John Trenchard Kn' one of our Principall Secre-
taries of State and Edw' Ruffell Efq'' our firft Commiffioner
for executing the office of our High Admirall of England,
Admirall of our Navy Royall and our Treafurer for the
fame, and our right trufty and well beloved S' Stephen Fox
Knight one of the Commiffioners of our Treafury, S' John
Lowther of Whit haven Baronett one of the Commiffioners
for executing the Office of our high Admirall, S' W'' Afhurft
Knight Mayor of our City of London, S' Robert Clayton
Knight, Sir Patience Ward Knight Sir John Moor Knight
& Sir W''' Pritchard Knight.

of Ground in Eaft Greenwich. All that piece or parcell of Ground fituate lying and
being within the parifh of Eaft Greenwich in the faid
Defcription of the Parcels. County of Kent and being parcell or reputed parcell of our
Mannor of Eaft Greenwich aforefaid containing in the
whole by Admeafurement eight Acres two roods and 32
Square perches be the fame more or leffe as the faid Ground
is now marke'd ftaked or otherwife fet outt. In which
admea-

admeasurem⁺ the Ground defigne'd for a way or paffage to lead thorow the premifes and herein aftermentioned to be excepted is comprehended or reckoned Which faid piece or parcell of Ground is bounded with our River of Thames towards the North and containes by Admeafurem⁺ along by the s⁴ River from the Tenement there late in the occupation of Nicholas Smithys or his Affignes to the Eaft End of the Edifice called the veftry there fix hundred feventy three feet of Affize be the fame more or leffe, and the s⁴ piece or parcell of Ground abutts in part on the publique Way leading from the Crane there to the Lane called the back Lane towards the Eaft and containeth towards the faid publique way three hundred fiftie eight feet of Affize be the fame more or leffe, and then returnes more Eaftward 72 feet of Affize litle more or leffe And then the s⁴ piece or parcell of Ground abutts in other part towards the Eaft upon the s⁴ Lane called the Back Lane and containes by Admea-furement ag⁴ the s⁴ back Lane one hundred ninety nine feet of Affize litle more or leffe, And the s⁴ piece or parcell of Ground from Eaft to Weft towards the South containes by Admeafurem⁺ fix hundred fiftie eight feet of Affize more or leffe including the thicknefs of the Brick Walls on both fides and doth abutt towards the South upon part of the ground of the old Tilt-yard and upon part of the Garden called the Queen's Garden the North Ends of the Ground of the old Tilt yard and of the s⁴ Garden and ab⁺ halfe the Edifice there now ufed for the fervice of our Ordinance being comprehended within thefe dimenfions as part of the Ground thereby intended to be paffed, And the faid piece or parcell of Ground towards the Weft containes in length from North to South by admeafurem⁺ feaven hundred and

eighteen

fors to the Intent neverthelefle that the aforefaid Premifes and every Part thereof ſhall be converted & imployed unto and for the Uſe & Service of ſuch an Hoſpitall as aforefaid, and that as ſoon as the Buildings thereof ſhall be finiſhed & that wee our Heires or Succeſſors ſhall create and eſtabliſh a Corporation or Body Politique for the Government of the ſaid Hoſpital and the revenues thereof that then the ſaid Sʳ John Somers Thomas Duke of Leeds Thomas Earle of Pembrooke & Montgomery Charles Duke of Shrewſbury Sidney Lord Godolphin Sʳ John Trenchard Eᵈ Ruſſell Sʳ Stephen Fox Sʳ John Lowther Sʳ Wm Aſhurſt Sʳ Robᵗ Clayton Sʳ Patience Ward Sʳ John Moor and Sʳ Wᵐ Pritchard and the Survivors and Survivor of them his & their Heires and Aſſignes doe and ſhall by the Command or Appointment of us our Heires or Succeſſors convey the ſᵈ Premifes and all their Eſtate therein unto ſuch Body Po-litique & their Succeſſors for ever. To be ſubject to ſuch orders Statutes Rules Conſtitutions & Appointments as Wee our Heires or Succeſſors by Letters Patents under the great Seale of England ſhall be pleaſed to make or eſtabliſh for or concerning the Foundation Rule & good Government of the ſaid Hoſpitall & the Revenues and Poſſeſſions of the fame and to & for none other uſe Intent or Purpoſe whatſoever. Provided always and we doe hereby promiſe grant & declare that the ſaid Sʳ John Somers Thomas Duke of Leeds Thomas Earle of Pembrooke and Montgomery Charles Duke of Shrewſbury Sidney Lord Godolphin Sʳ John Trenchard Edward Ruſſel Sʳ Stephen Fox Sʳ John Lowther Sir William Aſhurſt Sir Robert Clayton Sir Patience Ward Sir John Moor and Sir William Pritchard their Heires and Aſſignes ſhall from Time to Time by or out of the Profitts of the

Premifes

Premifes be reimburfed all fuch Charges and Expences as they or any of them fhall be neceffarily put to in the Execution of the Truft hereby repofed in them. And Laftly our Will and Pleafure is and Wee do hereby for us our Heires and Succeffors grant and declare that thefe our Letters Patents & every Article Claufe Matter and Thing therein contained fhall be good valid firme & effectual in the Law according to the true Intent and meaning of the fame and fhall be foe conftrued adjudged and taken in all our Courts of Record and elfewhere any Matter Caufe or Thing whatfoever to the contrary notwithftanding. In Witneffe whereof wee have caufed thefe our Letters to be made Patents Witneffe ourfelves at Weftminfter the five and twentieth of October in the fixth year of our Reigne by Writt of privy Seale.

Grant good in Law, &c.

Pigott.

' Copy

Copy of King WILLIAM's COMMISSION.

Tertia Pars PATEN de Anno RR. GULIELMI tertii SEPTIMO.

D. Comiss.
Georgio Principi
Danie et al
de Erectione
Hospital apud
Grcenwich.
(2)

WILLIAM the Third by the Grace of God, &c. To our dearly beloved Brother in Law Prince George Hereditary of Denmark The most Reverend Father in God Thomas Arch Bishop of Canterbury Primate and Metropolitan of all England and the Arch Bishop of Canterbury for the Time being our Right Trusty and Wellbeloved Councellour Sir John Sommers Knight Keeper of our Great Seale of England and our Chancellor of England Keeper and Commissioners of our Great Seale for the Time being our Right Trusty and Right Entirely Beloved Cousin and Councellor Thomas Duke of Leeds President of our Privy Councill and the President of our Privy Councill for the Time being our Right Trusty and Right Wellbeloved Cousin and Councellor Thomas Earle of Pembrook and Montgomery Keeper of our Privy Seale and the Keeper of our Privy Seale for the Time being our Right Trusty and Right Entirely Beloved Cousins and Councellors Henry Duke of Norfolke Earl Marshall of England William Duke of Devonshire Steward of our Household Charles Duke of Bolton Charles Duke of Shrewsbury one of our Principall Secretaries of State and William Duke of Bedford our Right Trusty and Entirely Beloved Cousins and Councellors John Marquesse of Normanby and Charles Paulett Esquire commonly called Marquesse of Winchester our Right Trusty

Names of Commissioners.

Truſty and Wellbeloved Couſins and Councellors Robert
Earle of Lindſey Great Chamberlaine of England Charles
Earle of Dorſett and Middleſex Chamberlaine of our Houſe-
hold Aubrey Earle of Oxford John Earle of Bridgwater
Thomas Earle of Stamford John Earle of Bath Daniell
Earle of Nottingham Lawrence Earle of Rocheſter Wil-
liam Earle of Portland Thomas Earle of Fauconberg
Charles Earle of Monmouth Ralph Earle of Mountague
Richard Earle of Scarborough Francis Earle of Bradford
Henry Earle of Romney Maſter of our Ordnance and the
Maſter of our Ordnance for the Time being Richard Earle
of Ranelagh in our Kingdome of Ireland Paymaſter of our
Forces our Right Truſty and Wellbeloved Couſin and
Councellor Charles Lord Durſley commonly called Viſcount
Durſley Son and Heire Apparent of our Right Truſty and
Right Wellbeloved Couſin George Earle of Berkley The
Right Reverend Father in God Henry Biſhop of London
and the Biſhop of that See for the Time being our Right
Truſty and Wellbeloved Councellors Robert Lord Lexing-
ton Charles Lord Cornwallis Sidney Lord Godolphin Firſt
Commiſſioner of our Treaſury Henry Lord Capell Thomas
Lord Coningeſby in our Kingdome of Ireland Charles
Mountague Eſquire one of the Commiſſioners of our Trea-
ſury Chancellor and Under Treaſurer of our Exchequer and
the Chancellor and Under Treaſurer of our Exchequer for
the Time being Sir John Trevor Knight Speaker of our
Houſe of Commons and Maſter of our Rolles and the
Maſter of our Rolles for the Time Time being Sir Robert
Howard Knight Auditor of the Receipt of our Excheq;
Thomas Wharton Eſquire Comptroller of our Houſehold
Sir John Trenchard Knight our Principall Secretary of

State and our Principall Secretarys of State for the Time
being Sir John Holt Knight Cheife Juſtice aſſigned to hold
Pleas before us and the Cheif Juſtice to be aſſigned to hold
Pleas before us for the Time being Sir John Lowther of
Lowther Baronett Sir Henry Goodrick Knight and Baronett
Leuitenant Generall of our Ordnance Edward Ruſſell
Eſquire Firſt Commiſſioner of our Admiralty Treaſurer
of our Navy and Admirall of our Navy Royall Richard
Hampden and Hugh Boſcowen Equires our Truſty and
Wellbeloved Sir Stephen Fox Knight one other of the
Commiſſioners of our Treaſury Sir William Trumball
Knight one other of the Commiſſioners of our Treaſury,
John Smith Eſquire one other of the Commiſſioners of our
Treaſury and the Treaſurer of England Treaſurer of our
Exchequer and Commiſſioners of our Treaſury for the
Time being Sir John Lowther of Whitehaven Baronett
Henry Preiſtman Eſquire Robert Auſten Eſquire Sir Ro-
bert Rich Knight and Baronett Sir George Rooke and Sir
John Houblon Knightes (which ſix laſt mencioned are
alſoe Commiſſioners of our Admiralty) and the High Ad-
mirall of England or the Commiſſioners for executing the
Office of High Admirall of England for the Time being
Our Right Truſty and Right Wellbeloved Couſins William
Earle of Craven Charles Bodvile Earle of Radnor George
Earle of Berkley and Arthur Earle of Torrington Our
Truſty and Wellbeloved Sir William Gregory Knight Sir
Giles Eyre Knight and Samuell Eyre Juſtices aſſigned to
hold Pleas before us and the Juſtices to be aſſigned to hold
Pleas before us for the Time being Sir George Treby
Knight Cheife Juſtice of our Court of Common Pleas Sir
Edward Nevill Knight Sir Thomas Rokeby Knight and

Sir

Sir John Powell Knight Juftices of our Court of Common
Pleas and the Cheife Juftice and Juftices of the fame Court
for the Time being Sir Nicholas Lechmere Knight Sir
John Turton Knight Sir John Powell Knight Barons and
George Bradbury Efquire Curfitor Baron of our Court of
Exchequer and the Cheife Baron Barons of the Coife and
Curfitor Baron of our Court of Exchequer for the Time
being The moft Revered Father in God John Arch Bifhop
of York Primate and Metropolitan of England and the
Arch Bifhop of Yorke for the Time being The Right Re-
verend Fathers in God Nathaniell Bifhop of Durefme Peter
Bifhop of Winchefter William Bifhop of Litchfield and
Coventry William Bifhop of Llandaffe Edward Bifhop of
St. Afaph Thomas Bifhop of Rochefter Thomas Bifhop
of Carlifle Jonathan Bifhop of Exon Thomas Bifhop of
St. Davides Gilbert Bifhop of Sarum Humphry Bifhop
of Bangor Edward Bifhop of Worcefter Simon Bifhop of
Ely Gilbert Bifhop of Hereford Nicholas Bifhop of Chefter
John Bifhop of Oxford John Bifhop of Norwich Richard
Bifhop of Peterborow Edward Bifhop of Gloucefter Robert
Bifhop of Chichefter Richard Bifhop of Bath and Welles
John Bifhop of Briftoll and James Bifhop of Lincolne and
the feverall Bifhops of the fame Sees for the Time being
Our Trufty and Wellbeloved Sir Edward Ward Knight our
Attorney Generall Sir Thomas Trevor Knight our Sollicitor
Generall Samuell Travers Efquire Surveyor Generall of our
Landes Sir Chriftopher Wrenn Knight Surveyor Generall
of our Workes Our Trufty and Wellbeloved Sir Thomas
Lane Knight Mayor of our City of London and the
Mayor of the fame City for the Time being Sir Robert
Clayton Sir Patience Ward Sir John Moor Sir William

C 2   Pritchard

Pritchard Sir Robert Jeffery Sir Thomas Stamp Sir John
Fleet Sir William Afhurft Sir Jonathan Raymond Sir Peter
Daniel Sir Samuell Dafhwood Sir Thomas Kenfey Sir John
Parfons Sir Edward Clarke Sir Humphry Edwin Sir Francis
Child Sir Richard Levett Sir William Gore Sir Thomas
Cooke Sir James Houblon Sir Thomas Abney Sir William
Hedges Knightes Thomas Darwin and Jofeph Smart
Efquires Aldermen of our City of London and all and
every the Aldermen of the fame City for the Time being
Our Trufty and Wellbeloved Edmund Bowyer of Camber-
well Efquire Michaell Godfrey Efquire Sir Leonard Robin-
fon Knight Chamberlaine of London Sir John Morden Sir
John Bankes Sir Jofiah Child Sir Peter Vandeputt Sir Wil-
liam Ruffell Sir Jeremy Sambrooke Sir Gabriell Robertes
Sir John Foche Sir Henry Furnes Sir William Scawen Sir
Jofeph Herne Knightes Sir Richard Onflow Baronett John
Lock Gilbert Heathcott and Arthur Shallett Efquires
Our Trufty and Wellbeloved Sir Richard Haddocke Sir
Cloudefley Shovell Knightes Edmund Dummer Charles
Sergifon Samuel Pett Thomas Willfhaw Dennis Liddall
Benjamin Timewell Efquires Principall Officers of our
Navy and the Principall Officers in the Nature of Commif-
fioners of our Navy for the Time being and our Trufty and
Wellbeloved Sir Charles Hedges Knight Judge of our Su-
preme Court of Admiralty Henry Guy Efquire Thomas
Pavillon Efquire Thomas Wefterne Efquire Charles Dun-
comb Efquire Peter Houblon Efquire Edmund Bolter
Efquire Thomas Firmin and William Lowndes Gentleman
Our Trufty and Well Beloved John Hill Efquire Mafter
and Affiftant of Trinity Houfe of Deptford Strond Captain
Samuell Rutter Captain John Bowers Captain John Conaway
Captain

Captain Roger Paxton Captain John Benbow Sir Mathew
Andrews Captain John Nicholles Captain Ralph Sanderfon
Robert Lord Lucas Sir Henry Sheere Knight James Sotherne
Efquire Captain Robert Fifher Captain George Phenney
Captain Samuell Atkinfon Captain Henry Greenhill Captain
Henry Rifbe Captaine Balchazar St. Michell Captain
Humphrey Ayles Captain John Jacob Captain William
Cruft Captain William Gutteridge Captain John Haflewood
and the Mafter and all and every the Wardens Afliftantes
and Elder Brethren of Trinity Houfe of Deptford Strond
for the Time being Greeting **Whereas** wee are extremely Recital—Defire to promote the Naval Strength of the Realm.
defirous that the Trade Navigacion and Navall Strength of
this our Realme of England (whereupon the Safety and
Flourifhing State thereof doth foe much depend) fhould by
all proper Meanes be promoted and advanced **And Whereas**
wee are perfwaded that nothing will more effectually con- But nothing will more effectually contribute thereto than Encouragement to Seamen.
tribute thereto then the endeavouring by due and fitting
Encouragementes to encreafe the Numbers of Englifh Seamen
as well for the Strengthening of our Navy Royall and better
performeing the Navall Services of us our Heires and Succeffors as for the fupplying and carrying on the Occacions
and Bufineffe of our Merchantes and other our Loving Subjects interefted in Trade Commerce Fifhing Plantacion
Difcovery and other Affaires relating to Navigacion **And**
Whereas the Seafaring Men of this Kingdome have for a That the Seamen of this Kingdom have for a long Time diftinguifhed themfelves, &c.
long Time diftinguifht themfelves throughout the World by
their Induftry and Skillfullneffe in their proper Employmentes
and by their Courage and Conftancy manifefted in Engage-
mentes and Hazardes for the Defence Honour of their Na-
tive Country **And** nothing is more likely to continue this Nothing more likely to continue.
their Ancient Reputacion and to invite greater Numbers of

our

our Subjectes to betake themselves to the Sea then the *Their Reputation, and invite greater Numbers, &c. than making a competent Provision for Seamen,* makeing some competent Provision that Seamen who by Age Woundes or other Accidentes shall become disabled for further Service at Sea and shall not be in a Condicion to mainetaine themselves comfortably may not fall under Hardships and Miseries but may be supported at the Publick Charge **And** that the Children of such Disabled Seamen *their Widows and Children.* **And also** the Widowes and Children of such Seamen as shall happen to be Slain in Sea Service may in some reasonable manner be provided for and Educated **And Whereas** haveing frequently reflected on the Premisses since our Accession to the Crowne Wee have determined with ourselves *Determination to erect an Hospital.* to erect and establish A Hospitall for the Purposes aforesaid **And altho'** by Reason of the Expensive Warr in which wee have been and are at present engaged wee have not been able to carry on the said good and pious Purposes to such Effect as wee have desired **Yet** in Order to begin to put the same in Execucion Wee and our late most deare Consort *Revisal of Grant of 25th October to certain Trustees in Fee* the Queen **Did** by our Letters Patentes under the Great Seale of England bearing Date the five and twentyeth Day of October last past Give and Grant unto you the said Sir John Sommers Thomas Duke of Leedes Thomas Earle of Pembroke and Montgomery Charles Duke of Shrewsbury Sidney Lord Godolphin Sir John Trenchard Edward Russell Sir Stephen Fox Sir John Lowther of Whitehaven Sir William Ashurst Sir Robert Clayton Sir Patience Ward Sir John Moore and Sir William Pritchard and to your *of certain Lands* Heires and Assignes for ever All that Peice or Parcell of Ground scituate lying and being within the Parish of East Greenwich in our County of Kent and being Parcell or reputed Parcell of our Mannor of East Greenwich aforesaid

containing

containing in the whole by Admeasurement Eight Acres
Twoe Rodds and Thirty twoe Square Perches be the same Exd.
more or leſſe as the ſaid Ground is now marked ſtaked or
otherwiſe ſet out IN WHICH Admeaſurement the Ground
deſigned for a Way or Paſſage to lead through the Premiſſes
and therein mentioned to be excepted is comprehended and
reckoned WHICH ſaid Peice or Parcell of Ground is butted
and bounded as in the ſaid Letters Patentes is expreſſed
And all that Capitall Meſſuage lately built or in building by and capital
our Royall Uncle King Charles the ſecond and ſtill remaining Meſſuage.
Unfiniſhed commonly called by the Name of our Palace at
Greenwich ſtanding upon the Peice or Parcell of Ground
aforeſaid and ſeveral other Edifices and Buildinges and other
Thinges in the ſaid Letters Patentes mencioned Except as
therein is excepted **To the Intent nevertheleſſe** That the
aforeſaid Premiſſes and every Part thereof ſhall be converted To be converted
and employed unto and for the Uſe and Service of our Hoſ- ployed as an
pitall for the Releife of Seamen theire Widdows and Children Seamen, their
and Encouragement of Navigacion in ſuch Manner as is Children, &c.
therein expreſſed and as by the Letters Patentes aforeſaid
(Relacion being thereunto had) may more fully appeare
And as wee are fully ſatisfyed That the Erecting of ſuch
an Hoſpitall as aforeſaid will be of great Benefit and Advantage to this our Kingdome **So alſo** takeing into our
Royall Conſideracion that the conſtituting and eſtabliſhing Rules and Sta-
a Foundacion of that Nature and the Frameing of Rules framed.
and Statutes for the Governement thereof in ſuch a Manner
as may beſt anſwer what is thereby intended and deſigned
is a Matter of great Difficulty and ſuch as does require
mature Deliberacion and Advice **Know yee therefore**
That wee repoſeing eſpeciall Truſt and Confidence in your
known.

known Difcrecions Abilityes and Integrityes **have** nominated authorized and conftituted **And doe** by thefe Prefentes
nominate authorize and appoynt you the faid Prince George Hereditary of Denmark Thomas Arch Bifhopp of Canterbury and the Arch Bifhopp of Canterbury for the Time being Sir John Sommers and our Chancellor of England Keeper and Commiffioners of our Great Seale for the Time being Thomas Duke of Leedes and the Prefident of our Privy Councill for the Time being Thomas Earl of Pembrook and Montgomery and the Keeper of our Privy Seale for the Time being Henry Duke of Norfolke William Duke of Devonfhire Charles Duke of Bolton Charles Duke of Shrewfbury and William Duke of Bedford John Marquefs of Normanby and Charles Paulett Efquire commonly called Marqueffe of Winchefter Robert Earl of Lindfey Charles Earl of Dorfett and Middlefex Aubery Earle of Oxford John Earl of Bridgwater Thomas Earl of Stamford
John Earl of Bath Daniell Earl of Nottingham Lawrence Earl of Rochefter William Earl of Portland Thomas Earl of Fauconberg Charles Earl of Monmouth Ralph Earl of Mountague Richard Earl of Scarborough Francis Earl of Bradford Henry Earl of Romney and the Mafter of our Ordnance for the Time being Richard Earl of Ranelagh Charles Lord Durfley commonly called Vifcount Durfley Henry Bifhop of London and the Bifhop of that See for the Time being Robert Lord Lexington Charles Lord Cornwallis Sidney Lord Godolphin Henry Lord Capell Thomas Lord Coningefby Charles Mountague and the Chancellor and Under Treafure of our Exchequer for the Time being Sir John Trevor and the Mafter of our Rolles for the Time being Sir Robert Howard Thomas Wharton Sir John Trenchard

Trenchard and our Principall Secretaries of State for the Time being Sir John Holt and the Cheife Juftice to be affigned to hold Pleas before us for the Time being Sir John Lowther of Lowther Sir Henry Goodrick Edward Ruffell Richard Hampden Hugh Bufcowen Sir Stephen Fox Sir William Trumbull John Smith and the Treafurer of England Treafurer of our Exchequer and Commiffioners of our Treafury for the Time being Sir John Lowther of Whitehaven Henry Preiftman Robert Auften Sir Robert Rich Sir George Rooke and Sir John Houblon and the High Admirall of England or the Commiffioners for executing the Office of High Admirall of England for the Time being William Earle of Craven Charles Bodvile Earl of Radnor George Earl of Berkley and Arthur Earl of Torrington Sir William Gregory Sir Giles Eyre and Samuell Eyre and the Juftices to be affigned to hold Pleas before us for the Time being Sir George Treby Sir Edward Nevill Sir Thomas Rokeby and Sir John Powell and the Cheife Juftice and Juftices of the Court of Common Pleas for the Time being Sir Nicholas Letchmere Sir John Turton Sir John Powell and George Bradbury and the Cheife Baron Barons of the Coife and Curfitor Baron of our Court of Exchequer for the Time being John Arch Bifhop of York and the Arch Bifhop of York for the Time being Nathaniel Bifhop of Durefme Peter Bifhop of Winchefter William Bifhop of Litchfield and Coventry William Bifhop of Landaffe Edward Bifhop of St. Afaph Thomas Bifhop of Rochefter Thomas Bifhop of Carlifle Jonathan Bifhop of Exon Thomas Bifhop of St. Davides Gilbert Bifhop of Sarum Humphry Bifhop of Bangor Edward Bifhop of Worcefter Simon Bifhop of Ely Gilbert Bifhop of Hereford Nicholas

D

Bifhop

Bishop of Chester John Bishop of Oxford John Bishop of
Norwich, Richard Bishop of Peterborow Edward Bishop
of Gloucester Robert Bishop of Chichester Richard Bishop
of Bath and Wells John Bishop of Bristoll and James
Bishop of Lincolne and the severall Bishops of the same
Sees for the Time being Sir Edward Ward Sir Thomas
Trevor Samuell Travers Sir Christopher Wrenn Sir Thomas
Lane and the Mayor of our City of London for the Time
being Sir Robert Clayton Sir Patience Ward Sir John
Moor Sir William Pritchard Sir Robert Jeffery Sir Thomas
Stamp Sir John Fleet Sir William Ashurst Sir Jonathan
Raymond Sir Peter Daniell Sir Samuell Dashwood Sir
Thomas Kensey Sir John Parsons Sir Edward Clarke Sir
Humphry Edwin Sir Francis Child Sir Richard Levett Sir
William Gore Sir Thomas Cooke Sir James Houblon Sir
Thomas Abney Sir William Hedges Thomas Darwin and
Joseph Smart and all and every the Aldermen of the same
City for the Time being Edmund Bowyer Michael Godfrey
Sir Leonard Robinson Sir John Morden Sir John Bankes
Sir Josiah Child Sir Peter Vandeputt Sir William Russell
Sir Jeremy Sambrooke Sir Gabriel Robertes Sir John Foche
Sir Henry Furnes Sir William Scawen Sir Joseph Herne
Sir Richard Onslow Baronett John Lock Gilbert Heathcott
and Arthur Shallett Esquires Sir Richard Haddock Sir
Cloudesley Shovell Edmund Dummer Charles Sergison
Samuell Pett Thomas Wilshaw Dennis Liddall Benjamin
Timewell and the Principall Officers in the Nature of
Commissioners of our Navy for the Time being Sir Charles
Hedges Henry Guy Thomas Papillon Thomas Westerne
Charles Duncomb Peter Houblon Edmund Bolter Thomas
Firmin and William Lowndes John Hill Captaine Samuell
Rutter

Rutter ... n John Bowers Captain John Conaway Cap- tain R... xton Captain John Bendbow Sir Mathew Andrew... tain John Nicholles Captain Ralph Saunderſon R... Lord Lucas Sir Henry Shere James Sotherne Captain ... t Fiſher Captaine George Shenney Captain Samuell ...kiſon Captain Henry Greenhill Captain Balchazar ... chell Captain Humphry Ayles Captain John Jacob ... William Cruſt Captain William Gutteridge Captain John Hazlewood and the Maſter and all and every the Wardens Aſſiſtantes and Elder Brethren of Trinity Houſe of Detford Strond for the Time being to be our Commiſſſſioner for the Purpoſes herein after mencioned **And to the End** That our Royall Purpoſe and Intencion herein may the better take Effect Our Will and Pleaſure is AND wee doe hereby order direct and appoint that you do from Time to Time meet together at ſome convenient Place for the Execicion of this our Commiſſion **And** that at your firſt or ſome other Subſequent Meeting or Meetings ſo many of you as ſhall be then preſent (of whom any one or more of you being of our Privy Councill and any one or more of you the Commiſſioners of our Treaſury and any one or more of you the Commiſſioners for executing the Office of our High Admirall of England for the Time being to be three at the leaſt) doe conſider of ſuch proper and fitt Methodes as you ſhall Judge moſt expedient to be obſerved in executing the ſame **And** wee doe alſo by theſe Preſents authorize and impower you our ſaid Commiſſioners or any ſeaven or more of you (of whom any one or more of you our Privy Councellors and any one or more of you the Commiſſioners of our Treaſury and any one or more of you the Commiſſioners for executing the Office of our High Ad-

mirall

mirall of England for the Time being to be three at the

leaft) to call to your Aid and Affiftance fuch Perfons as you fhall think fitt to affift and advife you in the due and effectuall Execucion of this our Commiffion **And** out of your owne

Numbei (as often as you fhall judge it expedient) to appoynt and conftitute fuch and foe many Sub Committees for the better manageing and carrying on our faid Purpofe and In-

tencion in this our Commiffion **And** to inveft them with fuch Powers as you fhall think fitt to intruft them with pur- fuant to the Powers hereby given to yourfelves **And** to

revoake or make void the fame and to revive and make anew the faid Sub Committees fo often as you fhall think needfull as aforefaid **And** wee doe by thefe Prefents authorize and require you our faid Commiffioners or any feaven or more of you (of whom any one or more of you our Privy Councellors and any one or more of you the Commiffioners of our

Treafury and *any or* more of you the Commiffioners for

executing the Office of our High Admirall of England for the Time being to be three at the leaft) calling to your Af- fiftance our Surveyor Generall of our Workes and alfo fuch other Artiftes and Perfons as you fhall think fitt) to confider what Part and how much of the Structures and Buildinges now ftanding upon the Peices or Parcelles of Ground con- tained in our Grant above mencioned will be unfitt or not ferviceable for the Hofpitall hereby intended to be erected and

in what manner fuch of the prefent Structures as you fhall think fitt to ftand may beft be altered fitted and prepared for the Ufe and Service of the faid Hofpitall in order to reprefent the fame to us with all convenient Speed **And** wee doe alfo authorize and require you our faid Commif- fioners or any feaven or more of you (of whom three or more

more to be fuch as aforefaid) forthwith according to the beft
of your Judgmentes and Difcreccions to prepare one or To prepare Mo-
more Modell or Modelles of fuch Buildinges Workes Erec- dels of Buildings
cions and Conveniencies as you fhall think moft fitt and to be erected,
proper to be erected and made in and upon the Premiffes by
us granted as aforefaid for the Ufe of the faid intended Hofpitall with fuch Schemes or Draughtes as may beft explaine with fuch
the fame and with all convenient Speed to prefent fuch Modell Drafts as may
or Modelles to us for our Royal Approbacion And wee explain them.
do further hereby authorize and impower you our faid Commiffioners or any feaven or more of you (of whom three or
more to be fuch as aforefaid calling to your Affiftance our And with the
Attorney or Sollicitor Generall or any other of our Councill Attorney and
learned in the Law for the Time being or fuch others as you Solicitor General
fhall think meet) to confider of and prepare a Charter or to confider of
Charters of Foundacion of fuch Hofpitall And alfo fuch and prepare a
Statutes Conftitucions Orders and Ordinances as may be And alfo Sta-
proper for the Foundacion perpetual Management Order Rule for the perpetual
and good Governement of the fame and of the Poor People the poor People,
Officers Servantes and others that fhall be entertained in and &c.
about the fame and for and concerning all other Matters
and Things relating thereto and to prefent the fame to us for
our Royall Confideracion And Whereas the greate and
earneft defire which we have to fet about foe good and pious
a Work has engaged us to begin the fame at this Time altho'
by reafon of the prefent Neceffity of our Affaires wee cannot
advance foe confiderable Summes for the begining and carrying on the faid Work as wee doe defire and intend and by
God's Bleffing in Times of Peace fhall be enabled to doe
Yet neverthelesse as a further Inftance of our Princely
Zeale for advanceing the faid Defigne wee have refolved and
determined

determined and doe hereby declare and make knowne that
from thenceforth wee will yearely caufe to be iffued and paid
out of our Treafure at and upon the Feaft of the Birth of
our Lord Chrift in every Yeare or at fuch other Time in
every Yeare as fhall be defired by our faid Commiffioners or
any feaven or more of them the fum of two thoufand

Poundes for and towards the edifying perfecting and endowing the faid Hofpitall **And** to that End wee doe hereby for
us our Heires and Succeffors require the Commiffioner of our
Treafury and Under Treafurer of our Exchequer now being
and the Treafurer of our Exchequer and Commiffioners of
the Treafury and Under Treafurer of the Exchequer of us
our Heires or Succeffors for the Time being withou any
further or other Warrant to be had or obtained from us our
Heires or Succeffors in that Behalfe from Time to Time to
direct their Warrantes or Orders for the Payment of the
faid Yearely Summe of two thoufand Poundes as aforefaid
out of fuch of our Treafure of us our Heires or Succeffors as
fhall not be appropriated to other Ufes to the faid Treafurer
for the faid Hofpitall hereby appointed or to fuch other
Treafurer or Treafurers as fhall be appointed as herein after
is directed at the faid Feaft of the Birth of our Lord Chrift
in every Yeare or at fuch other Times in every Yeare as fhall
be defired by our faid Commiffioners or any feaven or more
of them as aforefaid during the Continuance of this our
Commiffion **And** having no Doubt but that great Numbers
of our good Subjectes will be difpofed to follow our Example
and will with great Chearfulneffe and Readineffe contribute to
the advanceing fo charitable a Defigne which befides the
Releife of fo many poor difabled and neceffitous Perfons
will prove of great Advantage to the Kingdome in the increafing

creafing the Navigacion and Navall Strength thereof by encouraging fitt Perfons to betake themfelves to Sea Service as
foon as our Royall Intencions in the Premiffes fhall be made
knowne **And** that their affifting us in the Building and
Endowing the faid Hofpitall will be moft highly acceptable
to us wee doe by thefe Prefentes authorize and impower you
our faid Comiffioners or any feaven or more of you **And**
Wee doe by thefe Prefents Give and Grant to you or any
feaven or more of you full Power and Authority to take and
receive from fuch of our good Subjects as fhall be pioufly
difpofed to contribute towards the erecting and endowing of
the faid Hofpitall All fuch voluntary Giftes or Subfcriptions
of or for any Summe or Summes of Money Goodes or
Chattelles or of any Eftate or Intereft in any Mannors
Landes Tenementes Rentes Hereditamentes or other Matters or Thinges whatfoever which any Perfon or Perfons
fhall be willing to give limitt appoint or beftowe for or
towardes the Building Furnifhing or Endowing of the Hofpitall aforefaid And for caufing to be collected and received
whatfoever fhall be given contributed bequeathed defigned
or appointed for that Ufe by the Handes of the Treafurer
that fhall be hereafter appointed to receive the fame
And to the End that our Intencion in the Premiffes may be
better known to our Loving Subjectes wee doe require you
to caufe Publick Notificacion of thefe Prefentes or the
Tenor or Forme thereof to be made in fuch Places or by
fuch Wayes and Meanes as you fhall think moft conduceable
to the Furtherance of the faid Charity **And** wee doe alfo
by thefe Prefentes authorize and impower you our faid Commiffioners or any feaven or more of you (of whom any one
or more of you our Privy Councellors and any one or more

Commiffioners may receive Gifts or Subfcriptions of any Money, Goods, &c.

or of any Eftate or Intereft in any Manor, Lands, &c. which any Perfon fhall be willing to give towards endowing the Hofpital.

of

of you the Commissioners of our Treasury and any one or
more of you the Commissioners for executing the Office of
our High Admirall of England for the Time being to be
three at the least) in case you shall find the same to be
necessary for carrying on the Designe and Intencion of this

May appoint Deputies to take Subscriptions, our Commission by Instrumentes or Writinges under your
Handes and Seales to depute and substitute such Persons as
you shall think fitt to entrust to take such Subscripcions as
aforesaid and to collect or bring in the Moneys which shall
be contributed bequeathed designed or appointed for the
Uses aforesaid to the Handes of the Treasurer or Receiver
Generall hereafter appointed and to displace or discharge
such Substitutes or Deputies or any of them and to appoint
others in the Place of them or any of them from Time to

and establish Order for charging the Treasurer, &c. Time as you shall see cause And to settle establish and
appoynt such Cheques Comptrolles and Orders as you shall
think necessary or safe for the full and due chargeing of the
Treasurer and Receiver Generall and also the said Deputies
Substitutes, and all and every other Person and Persons what-

with the Monies they shall receive. soever whoe shall receive or be chargeable with any Moneys
or other Profittes for the said Charitable Use or Purpose to
answer pay or account for the same And that our said
Commissioners or any seaven or more of you from Time to
Time as often as you or any seaven of you shall suspect or

Upon suspicion of Fraud, &c. doubt of any Concealment Fraud or any Deceitfull or Indi-
rect Practice in reference to any Moneys or other Thinges
subscribed contributed given bequeathed or appointed to the

may examine Witnesses upon Oath. said Use shall and may enquire thereof by the Examinacion
of Witnesses upon Oath (which you have hereby Power to
administer) or by any other lawful Wayes and Meanes
whereby the Truth of the Matters in all such Cases may
best

beft be knowne and to proceed thereupon with Effect **And**
our Pleafure is **And** wee doe hereby require and command
That you our faid Commiffioners or any feaven or more of
you do from Time to Time certify to the Comiffioners of ^[to certify to the Treafury the]
our Treafury now being or to the Treafurer or Commiffioners ^[Names of Sub-]
of our Treafury for the Time being the Names of the Per- ^[fcribers, with the Sums fubfcribed.]
fons Societies Bodies Politick or Corporate who fhall fub-
fcribe or contribute give devife or appoint any Moneys or
any Reall Eftate or other Matters or Thinges towardes this
Charitable Defigne with the Summes of Money Goodes
Chattelles Eftate or other Thinges by them refpectively
contributed given limitted appointed or devifed **To the End**
a perpetuall Memoriall may be made of fuch Welldifpofed
Perfons whoe fhall become Benefactors as aforefaid and
whereby the Treafurer or Receiver Generall may be charge*th* ^[Exd.]
with more Certainty in his Accomptes **And in Regard**
wee doe confide very much in the Ability and Faithfulneffe
of our Trufty and Wellbeloved John Evelyn Senior Efquire
Wee have nominated affigned and appointed **And** wee doe
hereby nominate affigne and appoint him the faid John ^[John Evelyn]
Evelyn Senior to be the Treafurer and Receiver Generall of ^[appointed Trea-furer,]
all the Monies and other Profittes which fhall be fubfcribed
contributed given bequeathed devifed defigned or appointed
to or for the Building Furnifhing or Endowing of the faid
Hofpitall or for any Matter or Thing relateing thereunto
To continue in that Truft during our Pleafure **And** in ^[during Pleafure.]
Cafe of his Death or Removall Wee doe hereby Give full ^[And upon his Death or Re-]
Power and Authority to you our faid Commiffioners or any ^[moval,]
feaven or more of you (whereof any one or more of you our
Privy Councellors and any one or more of you the Commif-
fioners of our Treafury and any or more of you the Commif-
fioners for executing the Office of High Admirall of England
E

for

for the Time being to be three at the leaft) from Time to

Time to appoint one or more fitt Perfon or Perfons to the faid Place or Truft of Treafurer and Receiver Generall And fuch Perfon or Perfons from Time to Time to remove or difplace as you fhall fee Caufe And our Will and Pleafure is That the Treafurer or Receiver Generall for the Time being fhall have full Power and Authority And he is hereby fully authorized from Time to Time upon the Re-

ceipt or Receiptes of any Summe or Summes of Money or other Profittes for the Purpofes aforefaid or any of them to give an Acquittance or Acquittances for the fame which fhall be good and fufficient Difcharges to all Intentes and

Purpofes whatfover And the faid Treafurer or Receiver Generall for the Time being in his Receiptes Paymentes and Accomptes fhall be fubject to fuch Infpeccion Examinacion and Comptroll as you or any feaven or more of you (whereof fuch as are before appointed for a fpecial Quorum to be three at the leaft) fhall eftablifh or appoint And wee doe hereby for us our Heires and Succeffors ftrictly command enjoyne and require that none of the Moneys or other

Thinges which fhall be given contributed devifed bequeathed defigned or appointed as aforefaid fhall be diverted iffued or applied or be in any wife applicable to any Ufe or Purpofe whatfoever other then to the Charitable Purpofes before mencioned or fome of them or to defray neceffary Charges relateing thereunto And to the End that the Building and Fitting of the faid Hofpitall may be carried on with as much Speed as is poffible Wee doe by thefe Prefentes give full Power and Authority to you our faid Commiffioners or any feaven or more of you (of which any one or more of your our Privy Councellors and any one or more of you the

Commiffioners

Commiffioners of our Treafury and any one or more of you
the Commiffioners for executing the Office of our High
Admirall of England for the Time being to be three at the
leaft) when and as foon after as wee fhall have approved
under our Signe Manuall your Report or Certificate in that
Behalfe to take downe and demolifh or caufe to be taken
downe and demolifhed foe much of the Buildinges and
Structures nowe ftandinge upon the Ground by us granted
as aforefaid as fhall be judged as aforefaid to be unfitt or
not ferviceable for the Ufe of the Hofpitall hereby intended
as alfoe to convert alter and fitt fuch of the prefent Structures
as fhall be appointed to ftand as aforefaid in fuch manner as
fhall be appointed as aforefaid **And alfo** from and after
fuch Time as wee fhall have approved and allowed of fuch
Modell or Modelles as you fhall have prefented as aforefaid
under our Signe Manuall or otherwife fhall have allowed or
approved of any Modell Scheme or Defigne for building
fitting or furnifhing the faid Hofpitall **To putt** in hand
carry on and finifh with fuch convenient Speed as the Nature of the Thing and fuch Moneys as fhall be in the Handes
of the faid Treafurer or Receiver will admitt the Buildinges
and Structures of the faid Hofpitall and of all the Offices
and Conveniencies belonging thereto and to furnifh the fame
accordingly **In the doing** of which you are to purfue fuch
Modelles Orders and Direccions as fhall be approved or
appointed by us under our Signe Manuall as aforefaid **And**
our Pleafure is That you fhall proceed in the faid Workes
in fuch Order and Method and by fuch Waies and Meanes
and according to fuch Rules and Orders as to you fhall
feem beft **And** that you fhall call to your Ayd and Affiftance fuch fkillfull Artiftes Officers and Workmen as you

Commiffioners after their Report is approved of, may take down fuch of the Buildings

as fhall be unfit for the Hofpital, and alter fuch Parts as fhall be appointed to ftand.

And after the Models, &c. fhall be approv'd, are to carry on the Buildings, &c.

according to fuch Models, &c. as fhall be approv'd by Sign Manual.

To call to their Aid fuch fkilful Artifts,

E 2 fhall

as they shall think fit. shall think fitt and to appoint to them severally their respective Charge or Businesse And that you our said Commissioners or any seaven or more of you (whereof any one or more of you our Privy Councellors and one or more of you the Commissioners of our Treasury and any one or more of you the Commissioners for executing the Office of our High Admirall of England for the Time being to be three at the And direct Payment leaft) shall by Warrantes in Writing direct the Issuing Payment Allowances and Expenditure of the Moneys or Profitts to be contributed given bequeathed devised or appointed as aforesaid to buy or pay for Timber Brick Stone and other for Materials, &c. Furniture, &c. Materialles and for furnishing the said Hospitall with Bedds and other Necessaries and Conveniencies and to pay necessary and Salaries, &c. and reasonable Salaries Wages and Rewardes to the said Artistes Officers and Workmen which shall be employed in the Building as aforesaid and to reward those who shall be necessarily employed in bringing in receiving paying or accounting for the Moneys of the said Contribucions and to defray all other Charges and Expences incident to the Execucion of this our Commission or any Part thereof in such Proporcions Manner and Forme as you shall from Time to Time judge reasonable and meet. And that you or To make Orders for safe keeping and issuing the Money, Provision, Stores, &c. such of you as are last mencioned shall and do consider advise agree upon and sett downe Particular Orders and Instruccions as well for the safe keeping of the Money from Time to Time to be brought into the Treasury and of the Materialles and Provisions from Time to Time to be brought into the Stores as for the Faithfull and Frugall Issueing out and disposeing of the same for the Publick Use intended and And to direct how his Books and Accompts shall be audited, &c. none other And to direct and appoint by whom and in what Manner the Bookes and Accountes of both shall be

from

from Time to Time kept comptrolled audited and allowed
And out of your owne Number and fuch other Perfons of ^{And may appoint} Sub Committees.
knowne Integrity and Ability as you fhall choofe from Time
to Time and as often as you fhall judge it expedient to
appoint conftitute and make fuch and fo many Sub Committees as you fhall think meet for the better manageing and
carrying on of the faid Workes and to inveft them with ^{for carrying on} the Werks, and
Power to make Contractes and to do any other Matters or ^{to make Con-} tracts.
Thinges which you fhall think fitt to entruft them with
purfuant to the Power hereby given to yourfelves **And** to
revoke and make voyd the fame and to revive and make new
the faid Sub Committees or any other when and as often as
you fhall find it needfull **And** you and fuch of you as are
laft mentioned are to advife treat confider and determine of ^{And to confider} and determine of
all other Matters Wayes and Meanes for the Advancement ^{all other Mat-} ters, &c.
of this ufefull and neceffary Defigne and to put the fame in
Execucion till the faid Hofpitall fhall be compleatly built
finifhed and furnifhed with all Thinges neceffary thereunto ^{till the Hofpital} fhall be finifhed.
And further wee doe for us our Heires and Succeffors de-
clare and grant to you our faid Commiffioners and every of ^{Commiffioners} accountable for
you that you our faid Commiffioners and every of you fhall ^{their own Acts} only.
be only accountable and anfwerable to us our Heires and
Succeffors for your owne refpective Receiptes Actinges and.
Doinges and not for the Receiptes Actinges or Doinges of
one another or of the Treafurer hereby appointed or to be
appointed **Provided alwayes**. And our Pleafure is **And** wee ^{Treafurer may} retain a yearly
do hereby direct grant and appoint that the faid John Evelyn ^{Salary of 100l.}
hereby appointed to be the Treafurer and Receiver Generall.
as aforefaid fhall and may during his Continuance in that
Truft for his Paynes and Service in the Execucion thereof.
have receive retaine and keepe out of the Moneys that fhall.

from

from Time to Time be in his Handes by Virtue or Meanes
of his Receipt the Yearly Sallary or Allowance of Two hundred Poundes of lawfull Englifh Money at the Four moft
ufuall Feafts in the Yeare by equall Porcions to commence
from the Feaft of the Annunciacion of the Bleffed Virgin
Mary one thoufand fix hundred ninety five and to be from
Time to Time allowed upon his Accomptes Any Thing
herein contained to the contrary notwithftanding **And** thefe
our Letters Patentes or the Entry Exemplificacion or Enroll-
ment thereof fhall be to you and every of you and all others
herein concerned a fufficient Warrant in this Behalfe **In
Witneffe &c Witneffe** ourfelf at Weftmʳ the twelfth Day
of March.

P. Bre de Privato Sigillo &c.

**This is a true Copy from the original
Record remaining in the Chapel of the
Rolls having been examined.**

John Kipling

F A B R I C.

FABRIC.

IN purſuance of King William's firſt commiſſion, the Commiſſioners met at Guildhall, London, on the 17th of May, 1695, and appointed a Committee to view the piece of ground granted by King William and Queen Mary; which Committee reported that they were of opinion, King Charles's building then unfiniſhed, might, if an additional building ſhould be erected on its weſt ſide, be rendered capable of receiving conveniently between three and four hundred Seamen *(a)*. And at the ſame time deſired that the Lords of the Treaſury might be applied to for a Committee of Enquiry to reſtore and ſecure the water-ſprings and Conduits belonging to the ancient palace.

(a) Some perſons were of opinion at this time that it would be better to take down the wing erected by King Charles the Second as part of his intended palace, and begin the Hoſpital upon a plan entirely new. The diſputes on this ſubject ran very high, and it is reported that it had been mentioned to the Queen before her Majeſty's demiſe, and that ſhe was much diſpleaſed with the idea for ſeveral reaſons : 1ſt, That the expence of this palace was very conſiderable, and the materials after it ſhould be deſtroyed would not be equal in value to a quarter of the ſum it had coſt originally. 2d, That it was the work of Mr. Webb after the deſign of that eminent architect, Inigo Jones : and, 3d, That it was planned ſo as to correſpond with the Park which was laid out by Le Notre, a man of approved taſte. Several other places had alſo been propoſed for an hoſpital for ſeamen. Among others, the Caſtle at Wincheſter, but the preſent ſituation of the hoſpital was preferred, on account of its being ſo very conſpicuous and in the very ſight of London, to and from which port the great number of ſhips continually paſſing and repaſſing would afford conſtant entertainment to thoſe who had retired from the buſineſs of a ſeafaring life.

King

King William's fecond Commiffion having paffed the Great Seal in the month of September following, a general meeting of the Commiffioners was foon after held at Guildhall, at which were prefent

The Lord Mayor,	Sir Richard Onflow,
The Lord Keeper,	Sir Chriftopher Wren,
Mr. Stephen Fox,	Mr. Prieftman, &c.
Sir J. Lowther,	

When a grand Committee was chofen, confifting of fixty Perfons, to whom the immediate conduct of the Foundation was intrufted. This Committee firft met on the 23d of December following, and proceeded to refolve itfelf into three ftanding fub-Committees for the Fabric, the Revenue, and the Conftitution. Thofe for the Fabric were

Capt. Jonathan Andrews	Sir William Gore
Ant. Bowyer, Efq;	Sir Thomas Grantham
Wm. Bridgeman, Efq;	Wm. Glanville, Sen. Efq;
Capt. John Brumwell	Capt. Wm. Gatteridge
Sir Robert Clayton	Sir Richard Haddock
Dr. Salifbury Cade	Sir Jofeph Herne
Capt. Robert Dorrel	Sir Henry Johnfon
Wm. Draper, Efq;	Dr. John Mapletoft
Edmund Dummer, Efq;	Capt. Ralph Sanderfon
Thomas Fermin, Efq;	Sir Chriftopher Wren

The Preparation of King Charles's Building, and the erection of an additional one as before mentioned being the firft concern, certain powers for that purpofe were given to the Committee by the Co.i miffioners at a general meeting, when

when a plan of the intended alterations, which is preserved in the Record Room of the Hospital, was approved; and, being afterwards presented to King William, received his royal approbation also.

Before the Committee proceeded further, they fixed upon Mr. John Scarborough to be Clerk of the works, and Sir Christopher Wren, then the King's surveyor general, generously undertaking the conduct of this charitable work without any reward, the foundations of the new bass-building were laid in form by the Committee on the 3d of June, 1696.

This building being nearly compleated in 1698, Sir Christopher Wren submitted to the Committee a plan of a great dining-hall for the use of the officers and men (now called the Painted Hall) with an estimate of the expence, which meeting with the Committee's approbation, they ordered the ground to be set out for the purpose, and the work was prosecuted with so much industry, that the dome was erected, and the whole roofed in by the month of August, 1703.

In 1698 they also began to lay the foundations of the building, which answers to that of King Charles the Second, and is called Queen Ann's building; which name was given to it upon her Majesty's accession to the throne.

In 1699 great part of the foundations of the East Colonade and of the East Hall was laid.

F

In

In 1712 the north-weſt brick pavilion of the baſs part of King Charles's building was ordered to be taken down, and rebuilt with ſtone in ſuch manner as ſhould correſpond with the north-caſt pavilion of this building.

In 1725 the raiſing of the weſt front of Queen Ann's building was begun; and

In 1728 the ſtate of the ſtructure was as follows, viz. King Charles's building was compleated, except the ſtone pavilion at the ſouthern extremity of its baſs-building. Queen Ann's building, except the ſouth pavilion, had been raiſed and covered in.

The Colonades, with the porticos at their extremities, were compleated, and the whole of King William's building, which contained the hall and the weſt and ſouth dormitories, was alſo erected.

In 1752 Queen Mary's building, *(b)* in which is the Cha-

(b) On the 2d of January, 1779, a dreadful fire happened in the Hoſpital, which began in the north-caſt part of this building, and deſtroyed the chapel, with its dome, and part of the colonade. The conflagration was ſo rapid, that in the courſe of a few hours it not only conſumed the Chapel, &c. as aforeſaid; but alſo many of the wards adjoining.

Every means that could be deviſed was uſed to diſcover whether this misfortune was occaſioned by accident or deſign; but after a moſt ſtrict and diligent inveſtigation by the Directors, aſſiſted by Sir John Fielding, which laſted ſeveral days, and the offer of a conſiderable reward, nothing came out that could lead to a diſcovery.

An eſtimate of the expence of repairing the damages was then prepared, and orders were given for its being done with all poſſible diſpatch, beginning with the re-conſtruction of that part where the penſioners were lodged, which contained upwards of five hundred men.

pel,

pel, was finifhed, the rents and profits arifing from the Der-wentwater eftate having, in the year 1735, been affigned by parliament for that purpofe.

In 1769 a plan was approved, and afterwards carried into execution for rebuilding the fouth-weft brick pavilion of the bafs part of King Charles's building with ftone, to correfpond with the fouth-eaft pavilion of that building.

In 1778 the two fmall pavilions at the extremities of the terrace were erected and dedicated to their prefent Majefties.

Having thus traced the progrefs of this royal edifice from its foundation to this time, it now remains to attempt fome defcription of it in its prefent ftate.

GREENWICH HOSPITAL is fituated about five miles from London-bridge, on the fouthern bank of the Thames. It is elevated on a terrace about 865 feet in length towards the river, and confifts of four diftinct piles of building, diftinguifhed by the names of King Charles's, Queen Ann's, King William's, and Queen Mary's. The interval between the two moft northern buildings, viz. King Charles's and Queen Ann's, forms the grand fquare, which is about 273 feet wide.

From the entrance at the north gate, the eye, pafing thro' the grand fquare between the two colonades to the Queen's Houfe, is bounded by the Royal *(c)* Obfervatory erected on

(c) This obfervatory was begun to be erected on the 10th of Auguft, 1675, by order of King Charles the Second.

an

an eminence in the park; the whole prefenting the moft magnificent and beautiful *coup d' œil* that can be imagined.

In the centre of the grand fquare ftands a beautiful ftatue of his late Majefty King George the Second, executed by the famous Ryfbrach, and carved out of a fingle block of white marble which weighed eleven tons. This block was taken from the French by Admiral Sir George Rooke, and the ftatue prefented by Sir John Jennings, K^t at that time Mafter and Governor of the Hofpital, as a mark of his refpect and gratitude to his Royal Mafter. On the pedeftal are the following infcriptions by Mr. Stanyan* .

On the Eaft fide :
—— *hic requies feneĉlæ*
hic modus laffo maris & viarum,
militiæq;

On the Weft :
——*feffos tuto placidiffima portu*
accipit.

On the North :
hic ames dici pater atq; princeps

A N D

Underneath the royal ftandard :
Imperium pelagi.

* Author of the Grecian Hiftory, &c.

On

On the South :

Principi potentiffimo
Georgio 11do
Britanniarum regi
Cujus aufpiciis & patrocinio
Auguftiffimum hoc hofpitium
Ad fublevandos militantium
in claffe emeritorum
Labores———a regiis ipfius ante cefforibus
fundatum
Auctius indies et fplendidius
exurgit...

Jóhannes Jénnings *Eques*
Ejufdem hofpitii præfectus
Iconem hanc pro debitâ fuâ
Erga principem reverentiâ
Et patriam charitate·
pofuit
Anno Domini
MDCCXXXV

We now proceed to give a particular defcription of each of the four diftinct buildings before mentioned, all of which are quadrangular. The firft, called King Charles's building, is on the weft fide of the great fquare; the eaftern part of which was the refidence of Charles the Second, and was erected by Mr. Webb, after a defign of that celebrated architect, Inigo Jones; it is of Portland ftone, and rufticated.

rufticated. In the middle is a tetraftyle portico of the
Corinthian order, crowned with its proper entablature, and
a pediment. At each end is a pavilion formed by four correfponding pilafters of the fame order with their entablature,
and furmounted by an attic order with a balluftrade.

In the tympanum of the pediment is a piece of fculpture
confifting of two figures, the one, reprefenting *Fortitude*,
the other, *Dominion of the Sea.*

The north front, which is towards the river, prefents
the appearance of two fimilar pavilions, each having its
proper pediment fupported by a range of the fame Corinthian columns before-mentioned, and their entablature.
Over the portal, which joins thefe two pavilions, is an ornament of feftoons and flowers. In the tympanum of the
eaftern pediment which was part of the palace, is a piece
of fculpture reprefenting the figures of *Mars* and *Fame*,
and, in the frize, is the following infcription :

Carolus II Rex

A.REG XVI

The South front of this building correfponds with that of
the North, except the fculptures and infcription. The
weft front confifts of a brick building, called the *(d)* bafs-
building. In the middle it has a pediment with carving, in
the tympanum, confifting of the national arms fupported
by two Genii, with marine trophies and other ornaments.
The carving of the pediment is allowed to be well executed
in alto relievo; it is 30 feet in length, and 7 feet 7 inches in

(d) This bafs-building is intended to be taken down and rebuilt in a ftyle
fimilar to the reft.

height.

height. On the other fide of the fquare towards the Eaft,
is Queen Ann's Building, having its north, weft, and fouth
fronts nearly fimilar to King Charles's laft defcribed; but the
fculptures in the pediments, as well as in the weftern pediment of the north front of the laft-mentioned building ftill
remain unfinifhed.

To the fouthward of thefe are the other piles of
building, with a Doric Colonade adjoining to each. That
to the Weft is called King William's, and that to the Eaft
Queen Mary's.

King William's building contains the great Hall, Veftibule,
and Dome, defigned and erected by Sir Chriftopher Wren.
The tambour of the dome is formed by a circle of columns
duplicated, of the compofite order, with four projecting
groups of columns at the quoins. The attic above is a
circle without breaks covered with the dome, and terminated with a turret.

The weft front of this building is of *(e)* brick, and was
finifhed by Sir John Vanburgh, who was Surveyor of the
Hofpital. In the middle is a tetraftyle frontifpiece of
the doric order, the columns of which are nearly fix feet
in diameter, and proportionably high, with an entablature
and trygliphs over them, all of Portland ftone. At
each end of this front is a pavilion crowned with a circular pediment, and in that at the north end is a piece of
fculpture confifting of groups of Marine Trophies, and four
large heads emboffed reprefenting the four winds; with a
fea lion and unicorn.

(e) This part of the building is intended to be cafed with ftone.

The

The north and fouth fronts of this building are of ftone;
the windows of which are decorated with architraves and
impofts rufticated, and the walls crowned with cornices. On
the eaft ftands Queen Mary's building, in which is the chapel,
as beforementioned, with its veftibule; and a cupola correfponding to the other. Thefe two buildings were named in
honor of the Royal Founders, and were intended to have been
alike; but in the latter, however, more regard has been paid
to convenience than to ornament, and the whole front of it
is of Portland ftone and in a plain ftyle.

The Colonades adjoining to thefe buildings are 115 feet
afunder, and are compofed of upwards of 300 duplicated
Doric columns and pilafters of Portland ftone, 20 feet high,
with an entablature and balluftrade. Each of them is 347
feet long, having a return pavilion at the end 70 feet long.

The Eaft and Weft entrances of the Hofpital are formed
by two rufticated piers, with iron gates, having the Porters
lodges adjoining. On the ruftic piers *(f)* of the weft entrance are placed two large ftone globes, each fix feet in
diameter, one cœleftial, the other terreftrial.

☞ On the former are inlaid with copper, in a very curious
manner, twenty four meridians, the equinoctial, ecliptic,
tropics, and polar circles; and a great number of ftars of
the firft, fecond, and third magnitude, are reprefented ac-

(f) If thefe Piers and Globes were moved to the North Gate on the
Terrace adjoining the River (as hath been propofed) they would be feen to
muft greater advantage than in their prefent fituation.

cording

cording to their relative pofitions. On the latter, the principal circles are inlaid in the fame manner, with the parallels of latitude to every ten degrees in each hemifphere; the outline of the land and fea is alfo defcribed, with the track of Lord Anfon's voyage round the earth in his Majefty's fhip Centurion. The globes are placed in an oblique pofition, agreeable to the latitude of the place in which they ftand, and were delineated by Mr. Richard Oliver, formerly mathematical mafter at the academy at Greenwich.

In different parts of this extenfive fabric, commodious apartments are provided for the Governor and principal Officers, and wards are properly fitted up for the Penfioners and Nurfes; who (together with the Officers families, inferior officers and fervants, refident within the walls,) amount to nearly 2500 perfons.

When we confider the beauty, folidity, and magnificence of this fuperb ftructure, and the excellent ufes to which it is appropriated, it muft ever be contemplated with reverence and admiration, as a work of national grandeur, and at the fame time the nobleft monument of wifdom and benevolence.

The following Table fhews the names of the wards contained in each building, with the number of beds in each ward.

KING

KING CHARLES' BUILDING.	Gr. Floor.	1st Floor.	2d Floor.	3d Floor.
Monk . } weſt wing	11			
Prince . }	12			
Reſtoration } eaſt wing	8			
Orford . }	14			
Coronation } w.ſt		43		
Succeſs . }		11		
Neptune . . }			12	
London . . }			12	
Royal Charles . } eaſt wing		37		
Royal Eſcape and }				
Greyhound . }			18	
Soldado . . . }			12	
N. rth Crown . }			35	
South Crown . }			26	
Palliſer . ſouth wing				50
				301

QUEEN ANN's BUILDING.	Gr. Floor	1ſt floor.	2d Floor.
Jennings } . .		16	
Wager } weſt wing		16	
Edinburgh }		19	
Barrington } . .		19	
Auguſta } . . .		13	
Hawke . }		14	
Weaſel } eaſt wing		14	
Windſor- }			
Caſtle } . . .		16	
Royal- }			
George . } weſt .			40
Vanguard }			23
Victory . }			23
Weſt Norris } . . .			17
Prince of }			17
Orange . } eaſt .			
Princeſs of }			15
Orange }			
Eaſt Norris			15
Louiſa Hall . . .			10
Torrington . . . }			26
Cumber- } weſt .			
land }			24
Royal Oak			23
Shrewſbury . . .			17
Princeſs }			
Amelia }			15
Princeſs }			
Carolina . } eaſt. . . .			15
Hamilton }			15
Princeſs. }			
Mary }			15
			437

KING WILLIAM's BUILDING.	Gr. Floor.	1ſt Floor.	2d Floor.	3d Floor.
Boyne	48			
Naſſau	59			
Aſſociation and Kent .				
Hall		62		
Royal William		55		
Sandwich Hall		11		
Ramilies			50	
Barfleur			58	
Union . weſt wing . . .			46	
Marlborough				56
Namur				50
Britannia . weſt wing . . .				46
				551

QUEEN MARY's BUILDING.	Gr. Floor.	1ſt Floor.	2d Floor.	3d Floor.	4th Floor.
Sandwich	10				
Hardy	24				
Council	30				
Rodney	74				
Royal Charlotte . .		211			
Prince of Wales . .		82			
Anſon			76		
Duke			134		
Townſend			82		
Queen				210	
King				82	
New Ward					24
Duke of York					43
					1092

No. of Beds.

King Charles's Building . . . 301
King William's ditto 551
Queen Ann's ditto 437
Queen Mary's ditto 1092

Total 2381

R E V E N U E.

HIS Majefty King William in his fpeech to Parliament November 12th, 1694, faid, *(a)* " He would be glad they " would take into their confideration the preparing fome " bill for the encouragement of feamen; adding, that they " could not but be fenfible how much a law of this nature " would tend to the advancement of trade, and of the " naval ftrength of the kingdom, which was the great in- " tereft of the public, and ought to be their principal care."

A.D. 1694. 6 W. & M.

His Majefty fhortly afterwards granted 2000*l*. per annum towards the carrying on, perfecting and endowing of the Hofpital. And, incited by his gracious fpeech and encou- couraged by his munificent example, many individuals, confifting of the great officers of ftate and others chiefly of high rank, contributed alfo towards the profecution of fo laudable an undertaking, as appears by the following copy of the original Subfcription Roll in the poffeffion of the Hofpital, the preamble of which was drawn up by a com- mittee of the Commiffioners (confifting of the undermen- tioned perfons) at a meeting at Guildhall on the 31ft of May, 1695.

1694-5. 2000l. per Ann. granted by K. William.

(*a*). Journals of the Houfe of Commons.—Vol. 11th. p. 171.

The

The Attorney General, Sir Thomas Travers
The Solicitor General, John Hawles, Efq;
The Surveyor General, Samuel Travers, Efq;
  Sir Chriftopher Wren .
  Sir Robert Clayton
  Sir Patience Ward'
  Sir John Fleet
  Sir William Afhurft
  Sir Humphry Edwin
  Sir Francis Child
  Sir William Gore
  Anthony Bowyer, Efq;
  Captain R. Sanderfon
  Mr. Thomas Fermin.

" Whereas the King's moft excellent Majefty being ear-
" neftly defirous to promote the Trade Navigation & naval
" Strength of this Kingdom & to invite greater Numbers of
" his Subjects to betake themfelves to the Sea hath deter-
" mined to erect & eftablifh an Hofpital for all fuch Englifh
" Seamen & their Children as by Age Wounds or other
" Accidents fhall be difabled from further Service at Sea &
" for the Widows & Children of fuch as happen to be
" flain in Sea Service; In order whereunto his Majefty, &.
" our late gracious Sovereign the Queen's Majefty of bleffed
" Memory did by Letters Patents under the great Seal of
" England bearing Date the twenty fifth Day of October
" One Thoufand fix hundred ninety four give & grant
" unto feveral Truftees therein named their Heirs and Af-
" figns for ever for the Ufe of the faid intended Hofpital a
" Parcel of Ground in the Parifh of Eaft Greenwich in
          " Kent

" Kent with their royal Palace of Greenwich thereon erected
" by King Charles the Second and several other Edifices
" Buildings and other Things in the said Grant particularly
" mentioned: And whereas his Majesty by Letters Patents
" bearing Date the 12th Day of March one Thousand six
" hundred ninety four * hath nominated constituted and
" appointed Commissioners for the better carrying on his
" said pious Intentions & therein is pleased to declare that
" the present Necessity of his Affairs not permitting him
" to advance so considerable Sums towards the said Work as
" he desires; the Assistance of his good Subjects in it will be
" most highly acceptable to him, and therefore among many
" other Powers & Authorities to the said Commissioners
" given & granted, his Majesty has authorized and im-
" powered them to take receive and collect all such voluntary
" Gifts or Subscriptions of or for any Sums of Money
" Goods or Chattels and of or for any Estate or Interest
" in any Manors Lands Tenements or Hereditaments as
" any Person or Persons shall be willing to give limit ap-
" point or bestow towards the building or endowing the
" said Hospital His Majesty not doubting but that great
" Numbers of his well disposed Subjects will chearfully
" contribute towards this great and useful Design of pro-
" moting Trade and Navigation and encouraging the Sea-
" men of England who by their Skill & Industry their
" constancy and courage in all Engagements & Hazards for
" the Safety & Honor of their Country have from Time to
" Time signalized themselves throughout the World We
" therefore whose Names are underwritten do each for him-
" self subscribe and give for the Ends and Purposes aforesaid
" as follows.

* 1694-5.

I subscribe

I fubfcribe £. 500   Tho Cantuar*

500   J Somers C S

500   Leeds P

500   Pembrok C P S

500   Devonfhire *Ld. Steward of the Houfhold*

500   Shrewfbury *Secretary of State*

200   Romney *Mafter of the Ordnance*

300   Montague *Mafter of the Wardrobe*

500   Dorfet *Ld. Chamberlain*

500   Portland *Groom of the Stole*

200   Monmouth

200   Godolphin *Privy Counfellor*

100   Willm Trumbull K^t *Secretary of State & P. Counfellor.*

100   Chas Montague, Efq *Lord of the Treafury & P Counfellor.*

100   J Smith Efq. *Lord of the Treafury & Privy Counfellor.*

200   Fox K^t *Ld. of the Treafury*

100   Ranelagh *Paymafter of the Forces*

100   J Trevor K^t *Mafter of the Rolls & p Counfellor.*

100   J Holt *Ld Chief Juftice of England & p Counfellor.*

100   J Louther B^t *L^d of the Admiralty & privy Counfellor.*

100   H Prieftman Efq *Lord of the Admiralty*

100   T Lane K^t *Ld Mayor of London.*

100   R Auften Efq *L^d of the Admiralty*

100   Robt Rich B^t *L^d of the Admiralty*

                     I fub-

---

* Dr. Thomas Tennifon.

I subscribe £. 100 G Rooke K^t *Admiral of the Red, L^d of Admiralty.*

100 J^{no} Hublon K^t *Alderman of London & L^d of Admiralty.*

100 Geo. Treby K^t *Chief Justice of the com: Pleas.*

50 H Goodricke K^t *Lieu^t Gen. of Ordnance & p Counsellor.*

100 Patience Ward K^t *Alderman of London*

100 Wm Ashurst, K^t *Alderman of D^o*

50 Thos Rokeby K^t *Judge of King's Bench*

Marks

100 Edw Ward K^t *Chief Baron of Exchequer*

£. 0. Joh Powell K^t *Judge of C Pleas*

50 Sam Eyre K^t *Judge of King's Bench*

50 W. Gregory K^t *Baron of Exchequer*

50 John Powell K^r *Baron of D^o*

40 Littleton Powys K^t *Baron of D^o*

100 R, Onslow B^t *Privy Counsellor*

40 N Lechmere K^t *Baron of the Exchequer*

126 Richard Smith K^t *Baron of Exchequer*

40 H Hatsell K^t *Baron of D^o*

50 E^d Nevill K^t *Judge of the com Pleas*

40 Jo Turton K^t *Judge of the King's Bench*

40 Jo Blencowe K^t *Judge of the com Pleas*

40 H. Gould K^t *Judge of the K: Bench*

40 R. Tracey Esq *Baron of Court of Exchequer*

40 Tho. Barry Esq *Baron of Exchequer*

100 Tho. Trevor K^t *Ld Cheif Justice of com Pleas.*

I sub--

I fubfcribe £. 40   Ro. Price Efq *Baron of Exchequer*
                40   J. Smith Efq *Baron of D°*
                40   Ifaac Loader *of Deptford*
                20   Thomas Plume D. D. *Vicar of Greenwich*

A. D. 1695.
7 W. 3d.

The fecond Commiffion of King William having paffed on the 25th of September, 1695, his Majefty, in his fpeech to Parliament at the opening of the Seffion in November following, faid, *(b)* " that he had recommended to the laft " Parliament the forming fome good Bill for the encou- " ragement and increafe of Seamen, and that he hoped " they would not let this Seffion pafs without doing fome- " thing in it."

A. D. 1696.
7 & 8 W. 3d.

In confequence of his Majefty's Speech, an Act of Par- liament (called the Regifter Act) paffed this Seffion, by which it was enacted, that fixpence per man per month fhould be paid out of the wages of all mariners to the ufe of the Hofpital. And power was therein given to the Lord High Admiral, or Commiffioners for executing that office, to ap- point Commiffioners for receiving the faid duty.

A. D. 1698.
10 W. 3d.

(c) In 1698 his Majefty was pleafed to give to the Hof- pital one acre, two roods, and twenty-five perches of ground, lying contiguous thereto.

A. D. 1699.
10 & 11 W. 3d.

(d) In 1699, in confequence of an Addrefs from the Houfe of Commons to his Majefty, the Hofpital received a

(b) Journal of the Houfe of Commons, Vol. 11th. p. 339.
(c) Ditto, Vol. 13th. p. 54.
(d) Ditto, Vol. 12th. p. 600.

confiderable

confiderable pecuniary affiftance, his Majefty having been pleafed to give nineteen thoufand five hundred pounds, which were fines laid by the Houfe of Peers on certain merchants, fmugglers, as follows:

	£.
John Gaudet - - - -	1,500
David Barrow - - - -	500
Stephen Seignoret - - -	10,000
Nicholas Santini - - -	1,500
Peter Diharce - - - -	1000
John Peirce - - - -	1000
John Dumaitre - - - -	1000
—— Baudevin - - - -	3000
	£.19,500

And the fame year a Lottery was projected for the benefit of the Hofpital, which produced only fix hundred pounds. This Lottery was called the *Charitable Adventure*; and it was excepted by fpecial claufe out of a Bill for fuppreffing of Lotteries, upon petition *(e)* of the Truftees, afferting that they had demonftrated to the Archbifhop of Canterbury, the Lord Chancellor and others, that the Lottery would raife 10,000*l. per ann.* for the benefit of the Hofpital.

A.D. 1699, 11 W. 3.

By an Act paffed in the 12th and 13th of King William, it was declared and enacted, that it was and fhould be lawful

A.D. 1699. 12 & 13 W. 3.

(e) Journals of the Houfe of Commons—Vol. 12, page 657.

H   for

for his Majefty, his heirs and fucceffors to make any further
grant of grounds and lands, or edifices, lying near or adjoining to the Hofpital of Greenwich, as he or they fhould
fee neceffary, and think fit to give for the aforefaid ufe. —

A. D. 1700.
In 1700, the Earl of Romney affigned to nine of the
Commiffioners in truft for the Hofpital his grant of the
Market, (f) with a Court of Piepoudre thereunto belonging; and, in the year following, the ground where the market is now kept, and the Mews and other Edifices adjoining, were granted by the Crown to the Hofpital in per-
petuity.

A. D. 1701-2,
14 W. 3.
(g) In 1701-2, his Majefty was pleafed to grant to
Samuel Travers, Efq. Surveyor General and others, a
fmall piece of ground lying near the Hofpital, in truft for
the faid Hofpital.

A. D. 1705.
4 A. c. 12.
In 1705, the Hofpital received a gift from Queen Ann,
of the effects of Kid the Pirate, amounting to fix thoufand
four hundred feventy-two pounds one fhilling.

A. D. 1707.
In 1707, Robert Ofbolfton, Efq. by will, devifed
a large eftate to be equally divided between the two chari-
ties of Greenwich Hofpital; and the Corporation of the
Governors of the Bounty of Queen Ann for the augmentation of the Maintenance of the poor Clergy. A
moiety of which eftate (after paying certain legacies and

(f) This market is to be held weekly on Wednefday and Saturday.
(g) Journals of the Houfe of Commons, Vol. 13. p. 700.

                                                annuities

annuities) accordingly became the property of the Hofpital, and was valued at £.20,000. The unexpired term of his Grant of the North and South Foreland Lighthoufes, was a part of this benefaction : At the expiration of which term, a further Grant of them was made by the Crown to the Hofpital for ninety-nine years.

In the fame year, Prince George of Denmark, then Lord High Admiral, by his warrant gave a piece of ground in length 660 feet, and in breadth 132, lying on the Eaft fide of Greenwich Park, to be ufed as a Burial-ground for the Hofpital. And,

Anthony Bowyer, by Will dated November 3d, in the fame year, gave the reverfion of a confiderable Eftate of manors, lands, and tenements to Greenwich Hofpital, after the Eftate *En taille mâle* given to his brother Edmund Bowyer, Efq. and Sir William Bowyer, of Denham-Court, in the County of Bucks.

In 1708, by an Act of Queen Ann, as well as by feveral A. D. 1708. fubfequent Acts, the forfeited and unclaimed fhares of Prize 6 A. c. 13. and Bounty Money have been given to the Hofpital; and by an Act of the 12th, and another of the 22d of his prefent A. D. 1771. Majefty, authority is given to the Directors to caufe un- 12 G. 3. c. 25. claimed fhares to be refunded, in certain cafes therein men- A. D. 1782. tioned, for a limited time after they fhall have been paid 22d G.3. c. 15. into the Hofpital.

In 1710, by an Act of the 9th of Queen Ann, a duty A. D. 1710. was laid upon Coals and Culm, which was to be appro- 9. A. c. 22. S. 2 priated to building fifty new Churches, and towards finifhing

H 2 the

the building of Greenwich Hofpital and the Chapel, for
which purpofe £.6000 *per Ann.* was granted out of the
faid duty, which was afterwards continued for a longer
time by 5 Geo. 1ft.

In 1714, the General Court of Commiffioners and Go--
vernors having granted an increafe of falary to the Chap--
lains of the Hofpital, their wages, with the value of their
provifions and other allowances, as Chaplains of Woolwich
and Deptford Dockyards, were directed to be paid to the
Treafurer in aid of the Hofpital's Revenues.

A D. 1724.
11 G. 1.

In 1724, George the 1ft in his fpeech to Parliament,
expreffed himfelf to the Houfe of Commons in the follow--
ing manner *(h)*. " There is one thing that I cannot
" but mention to you as deferving your particular confider-
" ation : It is too manifeft that the funds eftablifhed for
" the finifhing the Works of Greenwich Hofpital, and
" providing for a compleat number of Seamen there, cannot
" in time of peace be fufficient to anfwer the expences of
" this great and neceffary work ; it is therefore very much
" to be wifhed, that fome method could be found out to
" make a further provifion for a comfortable fupport to our
" Seamen worn out in the fervice of their Country, and
" labouring under old Age and Infirmities."

The Commons in their *(i)* Addrefs promifed the King " to
" give every encouragement to Navigation, and to affift him
" in every thing that fhould tend to the fecurity and gran-

A. D. 1724.
11 G. 1.

(*h*) Journals of the Houfe of Commons.—Vol. 20, p. 331.
(*i*) Ditto,   Ditto, p. 335.

                                             " deur

" deur of his Majefty and his Kingdoms." But it does
not appear that any further provifion was made, 'till

In 1728, George the 2d in his fpeech (*k*) to the Houfe of
Commons after his acceffion, told them, " That he thought
" himfelf obliged to recommend to them a Confideration
" of the greateft Importance, and that he fhould look upon A. D. 1728.
" it as a great happinefs, if at the beginning of his Reign   1 G. 2.
" he could fee the foundation laid of fo great and neceffary
" a work, as the Increafe and Encouragement of our Sea-
" men in general; that they might be invited, rather than
" compelled by force and violence, to enter into the fervice
" of their Country, as often as occafion fhould require. A
" confideration, he faid, worthy of the Reprefentatives of a
" People great and flourifhing in trade and navigation. He
" then recommended to them the cafe of Greenwich Hof-
" pital, that care might be taken, by fome addition to its
" fund, to render comfortable and effectual that charitable
" provifion, for the fupport and maintenance of our Seamen,
" worn out and become decrepit by Age and Infirmities, in
" the fervice of their Country."

In confequence whereof, the Commons, before the end of
the Seffion, refolved for the greater encouragement of the
Sea fervice, that ten thoufand pounds fhould be granted in
aid to the funds of the Hofpital, which fum continued to   1. G. 2. f. 2.
be annually granted for many years afterwards.   c. 9, f. 9.

In the fame year, the Commiffioners and Governors
having fettled falaries on the Captains and Lieutenants of

(*k*) Journals of the Houfe of Commons, vol. 21, p. 22.

the

the Hofpital, the amount of their half-pay was directed to
be paid to the Treafurer, in aid of its Revenues.

And in that year, and for fome years afterwards, the Hofpital received a rent of about forty pounds a year, for fupplying feveral of the inhabitants of the Parifh of Greenwich with
water. This article of revenue has long fince ceafed, as
the Hofpital, on account of the encreafe of men on the
Eftablifhment, had occafion for all the water their fprings
could fupply.

A. D. 1730.   In 1730, a fmall piece of ground on the Eaft fide of
the Hofpital, clofe to the river, with a crane ftanding
thereon, which had been referved by the Crown in the
original grant, was given by his Majefty to the Hofpital.

In the fame year, Mr. William Clapham of Eltham,
by Will dated July 6th, gave to the Hofpital an eftate,
confifting of certain wharfs and warehoufes on the Eaft
fide of London Bridge, after the death of William Skrine,
Efq. and his fifter Elizabeth Crane, without iffue.

A. D. 1735.   (l) In 1735, his Majefty fent a meffage to the Houfe
S G. 2.   of Commons " recommending to them, to make fome pro-
" vifion for perfecting a work of fo much honor to this
" kingdom; and which had before received frequent marks
" of the regard of that Houfe."

Whereupon it was refolved in a Committee, (m) that the

(l) Journals of the Houfe of Commons.—Vol. 22, p. 432.
(m) Ditto,   Ditto,   458.

rents

rents and profits of the forfeited *(n)* eftates of the late Earl
of Derwentwater fhould be applied towards finifhing and
compleating the Hofpital; and when that fhould be effected,
towards maintaining the Penfioners; and an Act accordingly paffed for that purpofe, and for applying, in like
manner, the money which had been received on account
of the faid eftates, and then remained in the Exchequer, A. D. 1735.
amounting to 7182*l.* 13*s*; after paying the intereft and 8th G. 2.
arrears of the incumbrances then due: and to Lord Vifcount Gage 2000*l.* for his attention and trouble in difcover-
ing the fraudulent fale of this eftate, for which he received
the thanks of the Houfe of Commons, in 1732.

(n). The Rental of thefe Eftates was at this time about 6000*l.* per Annum,
encumbered with a mortgage of nearly 29,000*l.* and an annuity of 100*l.* the
whole of which incumbrances was difcharged by the Commiffioners in
1749.

By an Act of Parliament paffed in the 22d of G. 2d, 30,000*l.* was granted 22 G. 2.
for the relief of James Bartholomew Radcliffe, and the other children of
Charles Radcliffe, who was attainted for the Rebellion in 1715.

In 1775, the Commiffioners and Governors of the Hofpital were incorporated by Charter; and by an Act paffed foon afterwards, all the above 16th G. 3.
mentioned eftates were vefted in the faid Corporation for ever.

In 1788, in confequence of a petition from the Earl of Newburg, fon of
the above mentioned James Bartholomew Radcliffe, for the reftoration of the 26th G. 3.
above eftate on certain conditions; an Act paffed granting to his Lordfhip
and his heirs male a rent-charge of 2,500*l.* per annum, to be paid by the
Treafurer of the Hofpital.

In addition to the Public Grants and Donations above-mentioned; the following is a Lift of Benefactions to the Hofpital, from private Perfons, by Legacies or otherwife.

	£.	s.	d.
Sir Jofiah Child, - - -	300 :	00 :	0
Capt. Robert Bitton, - -	20 :	00 :	0
Brooke Bridges, Efq. - -	350 :	00 :	0
An unknown Hand in Malt Tickets,	1,000 :	9 :	8
Mrs. Thorold, - - -	50 :	00 :	0
Ralph Thurfby, Efq. - -	500 :	00 :	0
Thomas Blackmore, Efq. - -	100 :	00 :	0
John De la Fontaine, Efq. -	3,381 :	15 :	0
Benjamin Overton, Efq. - -	300 :	00 :	0
Sir James Bateman, - -	103 :	00 :	0
James Taylor, Efq. - -	102 :	11 :	5
Elizabeth Bridges, - - -	100 :	00 :	0
Mr. Evelyn, - - -	2,000 :	00 :	0
Mr. William Raphe, - -	250 :	00 :	0
Mrs. Waldron of Greenwich, -	500 :	00 :	0
Mrs. Waters, Widow, - -	100 :	00 :	0
J. Crofby, Efq. - - -	50 :	00 :	0
Admiral Long, - - -	100 :	00 :	0
Captain Sharman, - - -	100 :	00 :	0

	oz.	dwts.
Edmund Dummer, Efq. a Monteth and other Plate, containing	102 :	1
Captain William Sanderfon, Plate, -	65 :	1
Mr. Nicholas Hawkfmore, Plate, -	31 :	12
Mr. William Pate, and Mr. Abel Staney, Plate,	34 :	17

Dr.

	oz.	dwts.
Dr. Salifbury Cade, a large Tankard, &c.	65 :	1
Mr. James Thornhill, Plate, -	14 :	4
Rev. Dr. John Mapletoft, a Communion Service, - - - - } 96 :	14 gilt.
Mrs. Clements, widow of Lieut. Governor Clements, a Silver Tankard and Salver, } 39 :	6
Hans Hendrick, a penfioner, a Chalice,	18 :	2½
Captain Wm. Holden, a Silver Cup and Cover, for the fervice of the Chapel, } 21 :	9

We fhall conclude this Chapter with giving an account of the refpective fources from whence the whole Revenue of the Hofpital is at prefent derived, and alfo the principal articles of its expenditure.

R E V E N U E.

1ft, Sixpence per man per month for all feamen and marines belonging to his Majefty's fhips, including thofe in ordinary.

2d, Ditto for all feamen employed in the merchants' fervice.

3d, The duties arifing from the North and South Foreland Lighthoufes.

4th, The half-pay of feveral of the officers of the Hofpital who are entitled thereto.

I

5th, The wages, with the value of provisions and other allowances, of the two Chaplains of Woolwich and Deptford Dock-yards.

6th, The rents and profits of the Derwentwater estates, including lead mines.

7th, The rents of the market at Greenwich, and of the houses there and in London.

8th, Interest of money invested in the Public Funds.

9th, Fines for fishing in the River Thames with unlawful nets, and other offences.

10th, Forfeited and unclaimed shares of prize and bounty money.

EXPENDITURE.

1st, Cloathing, Victuals, Necessaries of all kinds, and weekly allowance of money to the Pensioners and Nurses ; together with salaries and allowances to the Officers and Clerks, and wages and allowances to cooks, scullery-men, and other inferior officers and servants.

2d, Ordinary works and repairs of the Hospital, including the Infirmary, Boys School, Brewhouse, and other buildings, and salaries to the officers, &c. in that department.

3dly,

3d, Contingent expences for Directors attendances, Law charges, stationary and various other articles, including the Derwentwater estate.

4th, Pensions to Out Pensioners including salaries to clerks, and other expences incident to that service.

The following is a Form by which any Benefaction may be legally bequeathed to the Hospital.

I A. B. do hereby give and bequeath unto the Commissioners and Governors of the Royal Hospital for Seamen at Greenwich *in the County of* Kent, *the Sum of*   *to be raised and paid by and out of all my ready Money, Plate, Goods, and personal Effects, which by Law I may, or can charge with the Payment of the same (and not out of any Part of my Lands, Tenements, or Hereditaments) upon Trust, and to the Intent that they do apply the same towards carrying on the charitable designs of the said Hospital.*

CON-

CONSTITUTION.

A. D. 1703.
Seven Commif-
fioners to com-
pofe a General
Court. By Queen Ann's Commiffion *(a)* dated 21ft day of July, 1703, feven Commiffioners were to compofe a General Court, whereof the Lord High Admiral, the Lord High Treafurer, or any two Privy Counfellors were to be a Quorum.

General Courts
to be held
quarterly. The Commiffioners were required and commanded to hold quarterly General Courts, which General Courts might alfo be called at any time, by order of the Lord High Admiral.

Officers to be
recommended
by the General
Court. They were alfo empowered and directed to recommend to the Lord High Admiral all Officers neceffary to be employed in the Hofpital; and his Lordfhip was empowered to appoint all fuch officers accordingly, except the Governor and Treafurer.

(*a*) This Commiffion was opened, and read at Windfor Caftle Auguft 17, 1703.   P R E S E N T,

His Royal Highnefs Prince George of Denmark, Lord High Admiral.
The Archbifhop of Canterbury.
Sir Nathan Wright, Knt. Lord Keeper.
Earl of Godolphin, Lord High Treafurer.
Thomas Earl of Pembroke and Montgomery, Lord Prefident.
John Duke of Buckingham, Lord Privy Seal.

Earl of Nottingham	Sir Thomas Littleton
Lord Granville	Mr. Draper
Sir George Rooke	Sir Chriftopher Wren

1

A ftanding

A ftanding *(b)* Committee, ftyled the *Directors* of the Hofpital, confifting of twenty-five perfons, were firft ap- Twenty-five Directors appointed. pointed by this Commiffion, who were commanded to meet once a fortnight at leaft, or oftener if neceffary, for the affairs of the Hofpital. They were made accountable for their proceedings to the quarterly General Courts ; and in confideration of their trouble and attendance, fuch as thought proper to demand it were to receive twenty fhillings each out of the Hofpital's revenue for every actual attendance.

By this Commiffion, either the Lord High Admiral, or Lord High Admiral or General Court to fill up vacancies of Directors. General Court, when affembled, were empowered to fill up vacancies in the Board of Directors.

It was likewife ordered that the government of the Hofpital fhould be performed by the Governor, and fuch a Government of Hofpital in Governor and Council. Council of the officers, as the Lord High Admiral fhould from time to time appoint.

(b) Names of the firft Directors : Charles Bertie, Efq; Sir Stephen Fox, Sir Henry Shore, Sir Chriftopher Wren, Sir Jonathan Andrews, Sir Mat. Andrews, Sir John Morden, Sir Thomas Grantham, Sir Francis Child, Sir James Bateman, William Bridges, Efq; Thomas Coulfon, Efq; James Craggs, Efq; Charles Godolphin, Efq; William Hewer, Efq; Robert Raworth, Efq; John Evelyn, Efq; William Draper, Efq; Edmund Dummer, Efq; John Vanburgh, Efq; Salifbury Cade, John Mapletoft, John Clements, William Sanderfon, Efq; John Brumwell, Efq;

Copy

Copy of the first Warrant appointing a Council.

His Royal Highnefs Prince George of Denmark, &c. Lord High Adniral of England, Ireland, &c.

To the Governor, Lieutenant Governor, Captain, three Lieutenants, Chaplains, Steward, and Surgeon, of her Majefty's Royal Hofpital at Greenwich.

" WHEREAS I think it fitting that fome perfons
" fhould be appointed to act as Council for the better ma-
" nagement of her Majefty's Royal Hofpital at Greenwich,
" and repofing efpecial truft and confidence in the ability,
" prudence, and circumfpection of you the faid Governor,
" Lieutenant Governor, Captain, three Lieutenants, Chap-
" lains, Phyfician, Steward and Surgeon; I do therefore
" hereby direct and require you, or any three or more of
" you, of which the Governor, Lieutenant Governor, or
" Captain, to be always one; to hold confultations, as often
" as need fhall be, and you fhall think proper for the good
" government of the aforefaid Hofpital; and to caufe to be
" executed the orders and punifhments prefcribed for fuch
" perfons as fhall be any ways diforderly therein; and to
" reprefent to me, as you fhall fee occafion, if any matter
" offer for my further directions therein.
" Given under my hand the 12th of July, 1705.
                        " GEORGE."
     " By Command of his Royal Highnefs,
         " G. CLARKE."

<small>Council ap-
jointed.</small>

                                     Several

Several other Warrants of the same nature have since that time been granted by the Admiralty, as the increase of Officers, or other circumstances have made it necessary. The present Council, appointed 11 March, 1774, consists of the Governor, Lieutenant Governor, four Captains, eight Lieutenants, two Chaplains, Physician, Secretary, Auditor and Steward.

The Council is held regularly every Friday, and oftener if occasion requires ; when Delinquents are punished either by mulct, wearing a yellow coat as a badge of disgrace, suspension, or expulsion, conformable to the Bye-laws for the internal government of the Hospital.

The powers with which the Commissioners and Governors, Directors, and Council, are invested, are set forth in the *Charter*, by which the Commissioners and Governors were incorporated, and of which the following is a Copy, viz.

C H A R-

C H A R T E R.

GEORGE the Third, by the Grace of God, of Great Britain, France, and Ireland, King, Defender of the Faith, and so forth, To all to whom these presents shall come, greeting. WHEREAS their late Majesties King William and Queen Mary did, by their Letters Patent, under the Great Seal of Great Britain, bearing date the twenty-fifth day of October in the year of our Lord one thousand six hundred and ninety-five, give and grant, to certain persons therein named, a certain piece of ground and a capital messuage within the parish of East Greenwich in the county of Kent, together with certain edifices, buildings, and other things in the said Letters Patent mentioned; to the intent that the same should be converted and employed unto and for the use and service of an Hospital for the relief of Seamen, their Widows, and Children; and an encouragement of Navigation, as therein mentioned. AND WHEREAS their late Majesties Queen Ann, King George the First, and King George the Second, did grant to several persons certain Commissions enabling them to erect and build an Hospital at East Greenwich aforesaid for the purposes aforesaid, and also granted several powers for the management thereof; BUT forasmuch as it hath been found that such powers have not been competent for the collecting, receiving, and applying the revenues, rents, profits, and emoluments given, appropriated, and belonging, or which may hereafter be given, appropriated or belong, to or to the use of the said Hospital, and

Recital of Letters Patent of William and Mary.

Recital of former Commissions.

Powers in such Commissions incompetent.

and have alſo been found inſufficient for other neceſſary and
beneficial purpoſes, whereby great inconveniencies and loſſes
have happened to the ſaid Hoſpital : To the end, therefore,
that ſo good and neceſſary a deſign, undertaking, and work
may be rendered effectual, and carried into better execution,
for the encouragement of Navigation and benefit of the
Realm, KNOW YE, that We, of Our eſpecial grace, certain knowledge, and mere motion, have willed, ordained,
conſtituted, appointed, and eſtabliſhed, and, by theſe preſents, for Us, Our heirs, and ſucceſſors, do will, ordain,
conſtitute, appoint, and eſtabliſh, that Our moſt dear brother
William Henry Duke of Glouceſter, Our moſt dear brother _{Names of the Commiſſioners and Governors.}
Henry Frederick Duke of Cumberland, the Archbiſhop of
Canterbury now and for the time being, Our Chancellor of
Great Britain now and for the time being or Our Keeper of
our Great Seal for the Time being, the Archbiſhop of York
now and for the time being, Our Preſident of our Privy
Council now and for the time being, Our Keeper of our
Privy Seal now and for the time being, Our Steward of our
Houſehold now and for the time being, Our Chamberlain
of our Houſehold now and for the time being, the Lords
and others of our Privy Council now and for the time being,
Our right truſty and right entirely beloved couſin and councellor Peregrine Duke of Ancaſter and Keſtevan Great Chamberlain of England and the Great Chamberlain of England
for the time being, Our right truſty and right well beloved
couſin and councellor Henry Earl of Suffolk and Berkſhire,
and Thomas Lord Viſcount Weymouth, and the right honourable Lord George Sackville Germain, Our Principal
Secretaries of State, and our Principal Secretaries of State
for the time being, the Warden of our Cinque Ports now

K   and

and for the time being, Our Treasurer of our Houfehold now
and for the time being, Our Treasurer of our Navy now and
for the time being, Our Master General of our Ordnance
now and for the time being, Our Lieutenant General of our
Ordnance now and for the time being, the Speaker of the
Houfe of Commons now and for the time being, Our Chancellor of our Exchequer now and for the time being, Our
Secretary at War now and for the time being, Our Master
of our Rolls now and for the time being, Our Commiffioners for executing the office of High Admiral of Great Britain and Ireland now being, and our High Admiral or our
Commiffioners for executing the Office of High Admiral of
Great Britain and Ireland for the time being, Our Commiffioners of our Treafury now being, and Our High Treafurer or Commiffioners of our Treafury for the Time being,
Our Chief Justice of our court of King's Bench now and for
the time being, Our Chief Baron of our Court of Exchequer now and for the time being, Our Chief Justice of our
Court of Common Pleas now and for the time being, Our
Justices of our Court of King's Bench now and for the time
being, Our Barons of our Court of Exchequer now and for
the time being, Our Justices of our Court of Common Pleas
now and for the time being, Our Attorney and Sollicitor
General now and for the time being, Our Judge of our
High Court of Admiralty now and for the time being, Our
Advocate of our High Court of Admiralty now and for the
time being, Our Secretary to our Commiffioners for executing the office of our High Admiral of Great Britain and
Ireland now being, and our Secretary or Secretaries to our
High Admiral, or our Commiffioners for executing the
office of our High Admiral for the time being, Our Secre-

taries to our Commiſſioners of our Treaſury now being, and
Our Secretaries to our High Treaſurer or Commiſſioners of
our Treaſury for the time being, the Flag Officers of our
Navy now and for the time being, Our Commiſſioners of
our Navy now and for the time being, the Maſter and the
five ſenior of the Elder Brethren of Trinity Houſe at Dept-
ford-ſtrand now and for the time being, the Mayor and the
three ſenior Aldermen of our City of London now and for
the time being, Our Governor, Deputy Governor, Treaſurer
and Receiver General, Auditor, and other Directors of our
Royal Hoſpital at Greenwich now and for the time being,
and the Surveyor-General of our Works now and for the ^{Declared to be one body politic}
time being, ſhall for ever hereafter be, by virtue of theſe ^{and corporate.}
preſents, one body politic and corporate, in deed and in
name, by the name of THE COMMISSIONERS AND ^{Name.}
GOVERNORS OF THE ROYAL HOSPITAL FOR SEA-
MEN AT GREENWICH IN THE COUNTY OF KENT;
and ſhall be Governors of the goods, revenues, rents, lands,
tenements, and hereditaments already given, granted, appropriated, or belonging, or which ſhall hereafter be given,
granted, appropriated, or belonging unto the ſaid Hoſpital.
AND We do, by theſe preſents, for Us, Our heirs, and ^{To have perpe-}
ſucceſſors, declare and eſtabliſh, that, by the ſame name, ^{tual ſucceſſion and a common}
they and their ſucceſſors ſhall have perpetual ſucceſſion and ^{ſeal.}
a common ſeal for the uſe of the buſineſs and affairs of them
and their ſucceſſors, with full power to break, alter, and ^{Power to break, alter, and make}
make new, their ſeal, from time to time, as to them ſhall ^{new their ſeal.}
ſeem expedient; and, by the ſame name, they and their
ſucceſſors, from time to time, and at all times for ever
hereafter, ſhall be a body politic and corporate in deed and
in law, and be able and capable to have, take, purchaſe,

K 2   acquire,

acquire, receive, hold, keep, poſſeſs, enjoy, and retain.

AND We do hereby, for Us, our heirs and ſucceſſors, give
and grant full authority and free licence to them and their
ſucceſſors by the name aforeſaid, notwithſtanding any ſtatute or ſtatutes of mortmain, to have, take, purchaſe, acquire, receive, hold, keep, poſſeſs, enjoy, and retain, to and
for the uſe of the ſaid Hoſpital, all or any manors, meſſuages,
lands, rents, tenements, liberties, privileges, franchiſes,
hereditaments, and poſſeſſions whatſoever, and of what
kind, nature, or quality whatſoever; and moreover to take,
purchaſe, acquire, have, hold, enjoy, receive, poſſeſs, and
retain, notwithſtanding any ſuch ſtatute or ſtatutes to the
contrary, all, or any goods, chattels, charitable and other
contributions, gifts, and benefactions whatſoever; and alſo
to ſell, grant, demiſe, exchange, alien, or diſpoſe of the
ſame manors, meſſuages, lands, rents, tenements, liberties,
privileges, franchiſes, hereditaments and poſſeſſions, goods,
chattels, contributions, gifts, and benefactions, or any of
them; and that, by the ſame name, they ſhall and may be
able to ſue and be ſued, implead and be impleaded, anſwer
and be anſwered unto, in all or any court or courts of record
and places of judicature within this kingdom, in all and
ſingular pleas, actions, ſuits, cauſes, matters, and demands
whatſoever, of what kind, nature, or ſort ſoever, in as large,
ample, and beneficial manner and form as any other body
politic and corporate, or any other our liege ſubjects, being
perſons able and capable in law, may or can have, take,
purchaſe, acquire, receive, hold, keep, poſſeſs, enjoy, retain,
ſell, grant, demiſe, exchange, alien, diſpoſe, ſue, implead,
or anſwer, or to be ſued, impleaded, and anſwered unto in
any manner whatſoever; and ſhall and may do and execute

all

all and fingular other matters or things, by the name aforefaid, as to them fhall or may appertain to do by virtue of
thefe prefents or otherwife. AND, to the end Our royal
purpofe and intention herein may the better take effect, Our
will and pleafure is, and We hereby direct, order, and appoint, that the members of the faid Corporation, or fo many
of them as conveniently can, fhall, from time to time,
meet together at fome convenient place, and they, or any
feven or more of them, fhall, and are hereby appointed to,
be a General Court, whereof Our High Admiral for the ^{To hold General Courts.}
time being, or any three of the Commiffioners for execut-
ing the Office of High Admiral now and for the time being,
Our High Treafurer for the time being, or any three Commiffioners of our Treafury now and for the time being, or
any three or more of the Lords of Our Privy Council,
herein before appointed Commiffioners and Governors, fhall
be a Quorum. And We do alfo by thefe prefents give and ^{Powers to finifh the building.}
grant unto the faid Corporation, or any feven or more of
them (whereof Our High Admiral for the time being, or
Our Commiffioners for executing the office of High Admiral now and for the time being, Our High Treafurer for
the time being, or our Commiffioners of our Treafury now
and for the time being, the Lords of Our Privy Council,
or any three or more of them, fhall be part) full power
and authority to proceed to finifh the building of the faid
Hofpital, according to the fcheme and model already be-
gun, or that fhall hereafter be thought fitting to be carried ^{To ftate the ac- counts, make payments, and manage the af- fairs of the Hof- pital.}
on ; and alfo to ftate the accounts for works of the faid Hof-
pital now and hereafter to be in hand ; to make payment,
from time to time, of the fame, and to direct, manage,
tranfact, conduct, and perfect all the bufinefs, affairs and

effects,

effects, matters and things whatsoever relating to the building, carrying on, and finishing the said Hospital, and the

To provide for seamen, either in or out of the Hosp.tal, their widows and sons. rents and revenues thereof; and also to provide for such Seamen, and such widows, and sons of Seamen, by pensions or
provisions issuing from the said Hospital, either in or out of
the said Hospital, in such manner and numbers, and under
such extent and limitations, as shall be thought necessary
and expedient and most conducive to the encouragement of
To execute leafes and make bye-laws, &c. seamen; and also to execute leafes for years, and make such
bye-laws, rules, orders, and directions for the better go-
vernment of the said corporation, as they, or the major
part of them so assembled, shall, from time to time, think
proper; which bye-laws, rules, orders, and directions, not
being repugnant to the laws or statutes of this Our realm,
shall be effectually observed, performed, and kept. PRO-
Bye-laws to be observed. Bye-laws not binding till confirmed. Method to be observed in repealing same. VIDED nevertheless, and Our will is, that no such bye-
laws, rules, orders, or directions, so to be made, shall be
binding, until the same shall have been confirmed by some
succeeding General Court; and that the same method shall
be, from time to time, observed in the altering or repealing
any such bye-laws, rules, orders, and directions, after they
shall have been so confirmed. AND Our further will and
pleasure is, and We do hereby require the members of the
said Corporation, or any seven or more of them (whereof
Our High Admiral for the time being, or our Commissioners for executing the office of High Admiral now and for
the time being, Our High Treasurer for the time being, or
our Commissioners of our Treasury now and for the time
being, the Lords of Our Privy Council, or any three or
more of them, shall be part) aforesaid, to meet and hold a
General Court to be held twice a year or oftener. General Court twice in the year, or oftener (if our High
Admiral

Admiral for the time being, or our Commiffioners for executing the office of High Admiral now and for the time
being, fhall find it neceffary) to confult concerning the bufinefs and affairs of the faid Hofpital, and the conduct and
management thereof; and that the Governor or Deputy- Governor, De-
Governor, Treafurer and Receiver-General, and Auditor of Treafurer, and
the faid Hofpital, now and for the time being, do affift at at all Meetings.
all General Courts and Meetings of the Directors of the
faid Hofpital hereafter mentioned. AND We do hereby Admiralty to
authorize and empower Our High Admiral for the time cers, except the
being, or our Commiffioners for executing the Office of Treafurer; and
High Admiral now and for the time being, to appoint all pend, or remove
officers neceffary to be employed in and for the faid Hofpital, haviour, and ap-
except the Governor, and Treafurer and Receiver General
thereof; and to difplace, move, or fufpend any fuch officer
or officers for his or their mifbehaviour, and to appoint any
other officer or officers in the room of him or them fo dif-
placed or removed. PROVIDED that all officers, to be
employed in the faid Hofpital, be feafaring men, or fuch All officers of
who have loft their limbs, or been otherwife difabled, in befeafaring men.
the fea-fervice. AND for that many of the members of
the faid corporation cannot conveniently meet, in order to
carry Our royal intentions in the premifes into execution,
and by reafon thereof many delays and inconveniencies may
enfue, We have thought fit, and do, by thefe prefents,
declare and appoint, that the Governor, Deputy-Governor,
Treafurer and Receiver-General, and Auditor of the faid Directors of the
Hofpital, now and for the time being, together with Sir Hofpital.
John Major, Baronet, *Timothy Brett*, Efquire, Sir *Merrik
Burrell*, Baronet, *Zachary Philip Fonnereau, Robert Pett,
James Stuart*, Efquires, Sir *Piercy Brett*, Knight, *John
Clevland,*

Clevland, Peregrine Cuft, John Tauzia Savary, Thomas Hicks, Efquires, Sir *Peter Denis,* Baronet, *John Barker, George Marfh, William Wells, William James,* Efquires, *John Cooke,* Clerk, and *John Campbell, Thomas Palgrave,* and *Joab Bates,* Efquires, who are the prefent Directors of the faid Royal Hofpital, fhall be a ftanding Committee, and be ftiled the Directors of the faid Hofpital. AND We do hereby give full power and authority, and require and command the Directors of the faid Hofpital now and for the

<small>To meet once a fortnight or oftner.</small> time being, or any five or more of them, to meet once in every fortnight at leaft, or oftner if occafion fhould require, to confult concerning the affairs of the faid Hofpital, and

<small>Secretary of the Hofpital, or his Deputy, to attend them.</small> that the Secretary of the faid Hofpital, or his fufficient Deputy, do attend at fuch Meetings. AND Our will and pleafure is, and We do hereby require and command the Directors of the faid Hofpital, that at all fuch Meetings

<small>Directors to take care to carry on the building.</small> they do take efpecial care of the carrying on the building of the faid Hofpital, purfuant to the model already begun, or that fhall hereafter be thought fitting to be carried on, and ftate the account for works of the faid Hofpital, now

<small>To ftate the accounts and make contracts.</small> and hereafter to be in hand, make contracts for provifions and all neceffaries for the faid Hofpital, and put and place out the fons of feamen, to be, from time to time, educated

<small>To place out the Boys as apprentices, not exceeding 7 years.</small> in the faid Hofpital, as apprentices, for any term not exceeding feven years, and do all other matters and things whatfoever relating thereto. AND We hereby give to the faid Directors, or fuch five or more of them, fo affembled, all

<small>General powers.</small> neceffary and fufficient powers for the purpofes aforefaid.

<small>Proceedings of Directors to be laid before General Court;</small> PROVIDED always, that all proceedings whatfoever, relating to the management of the affairs of the faid Hofpital, be laid before the General Court, to be held as herein

before

before mentioned, and the fame are to be at all times fubject
to their controul, to whom We do, by thefe prefents, give *and fubject to their controul.*
full power and authority to controul accordingly. AND
We do hereby order and direct, that the fum of ten fhillings
a man be paid to fuch of the Directors of the faid Hofpital, *Directors (fuch as demand it)*
as think reafonable to demand it, out of the revenues of the *to be paid ten*
faid Hofpital, by the hands of the Treafurer and Receiver *fhillings each for every attend-*
General thereof for the time being, for every actual attend- *ance.*
ance at every Board of Directors, and every General Court,
fo holden as aforefaid. AND Our further will and pleafure
is, and We do hereby give full power and authority to Our
High Admiral for the time being, or our Commiffioners for
executing the office of High Admiral now and for the time *Admiralty, or General Court,*
being, or the members of the faid Corporation affembled *may fill up the*
in a General Court, to fill up the numbers of Directors to *number of Di- rectors.*
twenty-four, including the Governor, Deputy-Governor,
Treafurer and Receiver-General, and Auditor of the faid
Hofpital, upon every vacancy by death, refignation, or refu-
fal to act, and to nominate fuch perfons as Our High Admiral for the time being, or our Commiffioners for executing
the office of our High Admiral now and for the time being, fhall think fit to be Directors in the room of fuch
perfon or perfons fo dying, refigning, or refufing to act, as
aforefaid. AND Our further will and pleafure is, and We *Governor, or any Officer except*
do hereby exprefsly forbid the Governor, or any other Offi- *the Directors,*
cers of the faid Hofpital, (other than the Directors afore- *forbid to make contracts, &c.*
faid, or fuch as they fhall appoint) to be concerned in pur-
chafing or making any agreement for provifions, or any
other neceffaries, for the faid Hofpital; or to have any other
powers, except the well government of the Houfe, and *Government of the Houfe to be*
even that fhall be performed by the Governor and fuch a *by the Governor and Council.*

L   Council

Council of the Officers of the faid Hofpital, as our High
Admiral for the time being, or our Commiffioners for executing the office of our High Admiral now and for the time
being, fhall from time to time appoint. AND we do hereby

authorize and empower the faid Corporation to take and
receive from fuch of Our good fubjects as fhall be difpofed
to contribute towards erecting and endowing of the faid Hofpital, all fuch voluntary gifts or fubfcriptions of or for any
fum or fums of money, goods, or chattels, or of or for any
eftate or intereft in any manors, lands, tenements, rents, hereditaments, or other matters or things whatfoever, which
any perfon or perfons, bodies politic and corporate, fhall be
willing to give, limit, appoint, or beftow, for or towards the
building, finifhing, or endowing the Hofpital aforefaid, and
for caufing to be collected and received whatever fhall be given, contributed, defigned, or appointed for that ufe, by the
hands of the Treafurer and Receiver General of the faid Hof-

for the time being. AND Our further will and pleafure is,
that the Treafurer and Receiver General now and for the
time being fhall have full power and authority, from time to
time, upon the receipt or receipts of any fum or fums of money, or other profits for the purpofes aforefaid, or any of them,
to give an acquittance or acquittances for the fame, which
fhall be good and fufficient difcharges to all intents and purpofes whatfoever; and that the accounts of the Treafurer and

Receiver-General of the faid Hofpital now and for the time
being fhall be examined, audited, adjufted, fubfcribed, and allowed, in fuch and in the fame manner as the accounts of
the prefent Treafurer and Receiver-General of the faid
Hofpital, and his predeceffors, have been heretofore examined, audited, adjufted, fubfcribed, and allowed, or in
fuch

fuch other manner as may, from time to time, be directed
by the members of the faid Corporation in General Court
affembled. PROVIDED always, and Our pleafure is, *Treafurer may*
that the Treafurer and Receiver-General of the faid Hof- *referve in his hands a yearly*
pital now and for the Time being, fhall and may retain and *falary of 200l.*
keep out of the moneys that fhall from time to time come
to or lie in his hands, as fuch Treafurer and Receiver General, the yearly falary or allowance of two hundred pounds
of lawful money of Great Britain, to be paid and retained *and the fame to*
quarterly, at the four moft ufual feafts in the year, by even *be allowed in his accounts.*
and equal portions, and to be, from time to time, allowed
in his accounts. AND We do hereby fully authorize and
empower the faid Corporation, at a General Court to be *General Court*
held as aforefaid, from time to time, to appoint and chufe *to appoint one or more receiver*
one or more fit perfon or perfons to be a collector or collec- *or receivers;*
tors, receiver or receivers, of the rents, revenues, contributions, or other profits and emoluments given or belonging
unto, or that fhall at any time hereafter be given or belong- *and may revoke*
ing unto, the faid Hofpital, and to revoke and make void *fuch appointments.*
fuch appointments as often as they may fee caufe fo to do. *Treafurer, and*
AND Our will and pleafure is, that the Treafurer and Re- *all other Officers entrufted with*
ceiver General of the faid Hofpital for the time being, and *money, to give fecurity.*
all and every other officer and officers, collectors, receivers,
or agents whatfoever, appointed or created, or hereafter to
be appointed or created, by Us, Our heirs, and fucceffors,
or appointed or to be appointed by the Lrod High Admiral,
or Commiffioners for executing the office of Lord High
Admiral as aforefaid, for the receipt or collection of the
rents, revenues, contributions, or other profits and emoluments as aforefaid, or any part thereof, or fhall be trufted
with the expenditure of any money for the ufe of the faid

L 2 Hofpital

Hofpital, fhall, within fuch time and times, as fhall be limited by the faid Corporation, give and execute fuch fecurity
for the duly accounting for and paying all money that fhall
come to their or either of their hands refpectively, on account for, or for the ufe of, or belonging to, the faid Hofpital, as fhall be thought fit and reafonable by the faid
Corporation, in General Court affembled, having regard
to the amount of the fum or fums of money that fhall be

All former com-
miffions (repug-
nant to this
Charter) void. ufually and commonly in their or either of their hands refpectively. AND We do, for Us, Our heirs, and fucceffors,
as much as in Us lies, determine, make void, revoke, annul
all and all manner of commiffions, charters, powers, and
authorities, at any time heretofore given or granted by Us
or any of Our progenitors, which any wife or in any kind
are inconfiftent with or repugnant to the grant, privileges,

Charter, or the
inrollment valid
and effectual,&c. powers, or authorities hereby given or granted, or intended
to be given or granted, to the faid Corporation. AND We
do alfo, for Us, Our heirs and fucceffors, grant and declare
that thefe Our letters patent, or the inrollments or exem-
plifications thereof, fhall be, in and by all things, good,
firm, valid, and effectual in the law, according to the true
intent and meaning of the fame, and fhall be taken, conftrued, and adjudged, in all Our courts or elfewhere, in the
moft favourable and beneficial fenfe, and for the beft advantage of the· faid Corporation, any non-recital, mif-recital,

to be fealed with-
out fine, &c. omiffion, defect, imperfection, matter, or thing whatfoever
notwithftanding. And that thefe prefents fhall be, in due
manner, made and fealed with the feal of Great Britain,
without fine or fee, great or fmall, to Us, in Our Hanaper

Promife of fur-
ther powers. or elfewhere, to Our ufe any ways to be rendered, paid, or
made. AND laftly, We hereby promife and declare, for

Us,

Us, Our heirs and fucceffors, that We and They fhall and
will, at all times hereafter, give and grant to the faid Corporation and their fucceffors, fuch other reafonable powers
and authorities as may be neceffary for the better execution
of the premifes. IN WITNESS whereof We have caufed
thefe Our letters to be made patent. WITNESS Ourfelf
at Weftminfter, the fixth day of December, in the fixteenth
year of Our reign.

By Writ of Privy Seal,

W I L M O T.

N. B. By an Act of the 16 Geo. 3. c. 24. all the eftates
held in truft for the benefit of the Hofpital, were vefted in
the Commiffioners and Governors incorporated by this
Charter.

ESTAB-

ESTABLISHMENT.

A. D. 1696.
7 & 8th W.
c. 21.

B_Y the Regifter Act of the 7th and 8th of King William the Third, it was directed that thofe Seamen who were duly regiftered, and who by age, wounds, and other accidents, were difabled for further fervice at fea, and could not provide for themfelves, fhould, upon certificate thereof, from the Captain, Mafter, &c. under his or their hands and feal, unto the Governor of the Hofpital, be admitted into the fame; and that the Widows and Children of fuch as

Admiffions re-
gulated by the
Regifter Act.
A. D. 1698.
8 & 9 W. c. 23.

fhould be flain, killed or drowned in the fervice, fhould be received into the Hofpital, and that the faid Children fhould be educated at the charges of the faid Hofpital, till they were fit to be put out, or of ability to maintain themfelves. And in the 9th of William the Third it was enacted, that the preference of admiffion fhould be given to fuch as had been the longeft regiftered.

But feveral doubts having arifen whether *any* difabled Seaman, otherwife than fuch as were exprefsly qualified by thefe Acts, might be admitted and provided for in the Hofpital; an Act paffed in the fecond year of Queen Ann, entitled, " An Act for the increafe of feamen," &c. whereby it was enacted, that *any* difabled Seamen, their Wives and Children, and the Widows and Children of Seamen flain, killed or drowned in the fea fervice, fhould

By the difcretion
of the Lord High
Admiral,
2 A.

be appointed and provided for in the Hofpital, as the Lord High Admiral, or Commiffioners for executing the office of Lord High Admiral, fhould think fit, or fee occafion.

By

By her Majesty's second Commission, dated the 8th A. D. 1704. Officers or others to be sea-faring-men. day of April, 1704, it was directed, that for the future, all perfons to be recommended and admitted into the Hofpital as Officers, or otherwife, fhould be fea-faring men, or fuch as had loft their limbs, or had been otherwife difabled in the fea-fervice.

By an Act of Parliament paffed in the 6th year of Queen A. D. 1707. Foreigners.. 6 A. c. 37. Ann, it was enacted that foreigners who had ferved for two years in her Majefty's fhips of war, privateer, or merchant-fhi, fhould be invefted with the privileges granted to the fubjects of Great Britain.

By an Act paffed in the 10th year of her Reign, any feaman A. D. 1710. Merchant Sea-men. 10 A. c. 17. in the merchant-fervice who had been difbabled in defend-ing or taking any fhip, as deemed qualified to be admitted into the Hofpital.

By the Act for the more effectual fuppreffing of piracy, A. D. 1714. 8 G. 1. c. 24. Seamen maimed in engagements with Pirates. paffed in the 8th year of George the Firft, any feaman who was maimed in fight againft any pirate in the defence of the King's or merchant-fhips, or any other fhip or veffel, was entitled to admiffion and provifion in the Hof-pital in preference to any other feaman difabled for fervice, or from getting his livelihood merely by age.

Having fhewn what defcription of perfons are qualified by the Commiffions, and the above Acts of Parliament, to be received into the Hofpital, we proceed to give an account of their admiffion from the firft eftablifhment to the prefent time.

On.

On the firſt of December, 1704, it having been repreſented to the Lord High Admiral by the Commiſſioners,
that the Hoſpital was prepared for the reception of men,
his Royal Highneſs Prince George of Denmark, previous
to their admiſſion, appointed the following officers by
warrant.

> A Lieutenant Governor
> A Captain
> A Firſt Lieutenant
> A Second ditto
> A Phyſician
> A Surgeon
> A Steward
> A Cook
> A Butler's Mate
> Four Nurſes.

And, in the month following he appointed

> Two Chaplains, and
> A Third Lieutenant.

In addition to the foregoing, the following Officers were
afterwards appointed, viz.

> In 1708, the Firſt Maſter and Governor
> 1736, a Second Captain
> 1738, a Fourth Lieutenant
> 1748. Fifth and Sixth Lieutenants
> 1756, a Third Captain
> 1766, Seventh and Eight Lieutenants
> 1767, a Fourth Captain.

We

We will now give an account of the admiffion of the
Penfioners, and their increafe from time to time as the
Hofpital was able to receive them; obferving at the fame
time, that, from the firft eftablifhment of the Hofpital,
Marines, as well as Seamen, if proper objects, were admitted
without any diftinction.

PENSIONERS.

In January	-	1705	- 42
From 1705	to	1708	- 258
1708	to	1709	- 50
1709	to	1728	- 100
1728	to	1731	- 450
1737	to	1738	- 100
1748	to	1751	- 300
1752	to	1755	- 250
From June to December 1763			- 170
From February to April 1764			- 63
1769	to	1770	- 217
1772	to	1782	- 350

Total 2350

M

Prefent

Prefent Eftablifhment of Officers,&c.

	Salaries. £.	Clerks and Affiftants.
A Mafter and Governor	1000	—1 Clerk at 50*l.*
A Lieutenant Governor	400	
Four Captains, each	230	
Eight Lieutenants, each	115	
A Treafurer and Receiver	200	—3* Clerks at 50*l.*
A Secretary - -	160	—2 Clerks, 1 at 60*l.* and 1 at 50*l.*
An Auditor - -	100	—1 Clerk at 50*l.*
Two Chaplains, each	130	
A Phyfician, 10*s. per diem,*	182 10*s.*	
A Steward - -	160	—4 Clerks, 1 at 60*l.* and 3 at 40*l.* each.
A Surgeon - -	150	—3 Affiftants at 40*l.* each, 1 fervant at 30*l.*
A Clerk of the Checque	160	—4 Clerks, 1 at 60*l.* and 3 at 40*l.* each.
A Surveyor - -	200	
A Clerk of the Works, 5*s.* per day	91 5*s.*	1 Clerk at 60*l.*
A Difpenfer - -	50	—1 Affiftant at 30*l.*
Three Matrons, each -	40	
A Schoolmafter - -	150	
A Mafter Brewer -	60	
An Organift - -	60	
A Butler - -	25	—2 Mates at 15*l.* each.
Two Cooks, each -	30	—4 Mates, viz. 2 at 20*l.* and 2 at 15*l.*

* One of them was appointed on account of Out-penfioners—and the 1ft Clerk has 50*l.* more on the fame account.

A Scul-

	Salaries.	Clerks and Affiftants.
	£.	
A Sculleryman	20	—2 Mates at 15*l*. each.
A Meffenger	30	
Two Porters, each	15	
Barber	12	

The Governor and Treafurer are appointed by Patent, the reft of the Officers by the Admiralty; except the Surveyor and Clerk of the Works, who are appointed by the General Court, the Schoolmafter and Meffenger by the Board of Directors, and all the Clerks by their refpective Superiors.

The Officers are allowed a certain quantity of coals and candles, and 14*d*. per day in lieu of a table with which they were originally accommodated; and moft of the under Officers are allowed provifions in the fame manner as the Penfioners.

There are alfo five days fet apart for Feftivals, viz.

THE ROYAL FOUNDERS CORONATION.

THE KING's BIRTH-DAY.

. . . . . . ACCESSION.

. . . . . . CORONATION.

THE QUEEN's BIRTH DAY.

P E N S I O N E R S.

The number of Penfioners now maintained in the Hofpital is 2350—every Boatfwain is allowed 2s. 6d; every Mate 1s. 6d, and every private Man 1s, per week for pocket money.

*C L O T H I N G.

A Blue Suit   ⎫
A Hat   ⎪
Three Pair of Blue Yarn Hofe   ⎬ In two Years.
Three Pair of Shoes   ⎪
Four Shirts   ⎭

The Coats and Hats of the Boatfwains and Boatfwains-Mates are diftinguifhed; the former by a broad, and the latter by a narrow, gold lace.

The Penfioners are alfo allowed Neckcloths, Nightcaps, and all neceffaries for bedding, which are changed as worn out.

Great Coats are allowed for the old and infirm, and Watch-coats for thofe on guard.

20 G. 2.

* *By an Act of Parliament paffed in the 20th year of George 2d, it was enacted, that perfons taking to pawn clothes belonging to the Hofpital, or changing the colour or marks thereof, fhould forfeit 5l. upon conviction before one of his Majefty's Juftices of the Peace; or be committed to prifon for three months: and that the Penfioner, or Nurfe, going off with the fame, fhould be committed for fix months. One moiety of this fum is directed to be paid to the informer, the other for the benefit of the Hofpital.*

T A B L E

TABLE of DIET.

Days.	Bread Loaves of 16 oz.	Beer Quarts	Beef lb.	Mutton lb.	Butter lb.	Cheese lb.	Peafe Pints.
Sunday	1	2	—	1	—	$\frac{1}{4}$	—
Monday	1	2	1	—	—	$\frac{1}{4}$	—
Tuefday	1	2	—	1	—	$\frac{1}{4}$	—
Wednefd.	1	2	—	—	$\frac{1}{16}$	$\frac{1}{2}$	$\frac{1}{2}$
Thurfday	1	2	1	—	—	$\frac{1}{4}$	—
Friday	1	2	—	—	$\frac{1}{16}$	$\frac{1}{4}$	$\frac{1}{2}$
Saturday	1	2	1	—	—	$\frac{1}{4}$	—
Total per Week	7	14	3	2	$\frac{2}{16}$	$\frac{1}{14}$	1

The Hofpital bake their own bread, and brew their own beer, for which purpofes commodious buildings have been erected.

The Penfioners dine at 12 o'clock, when the Lieutenant on duty attends to fee that good order be preferved during their meals.

N. B. The furplus of peafe-foup, being a confiderable quantity, is given away to the Penfioners families at the gates of the Hofpital.

All

Perfons defirous of being admitted penfioners, apply at the Admiralty Office, at leaft ten days before the day of Examination,* where they receive letters directed to the proper Officer at the Navy-office, for Certificates of their time of fervice in the Navy, which Certificates are fent to the Admiralty prior to the day of examination, when the Candidates are feen by the Board (the Surgeon of the Hofpital attending) and thofe who are found to be proper objects are minuted to be fent to the Hofpital, and are fent accordingly as vacancies happen; the greateft objects in preference.

N U R S E S.

The number now employed is 147; they are appointed by Warrant from the Admiralty, and muft all be Widows of Seamen; and under the age of 45 years, at the time of admiffion.

Their allowances are as follows, viz.
Wages, each, per annum, 8l.
A grey ferge gown and petticoat, yearly.
Provifions }
Bedding   } the fame as a Penfioner.

The Nurfes are required to take out Certificates of their hufband's fervice in the Navy in the fame mode as the Penfioners; and to produce Certificates of their age and marriage to the Admiralty on the day of examination.

About 14,000 Penfioners, and 600 Nurfes have been admitted into the Hofpital from its firft eftablifhment to the prefent time.

* The days at prefent appointed for that purpofe are the firft Thurfdays in January, April, July, and October.

The

The Establishment of Out-Pensioners.

On the 1st. day of February, 1763, the Commissioners and Governors, at an extraordinary General Court, took into their consideration the state of the revenue and expence of the Hospital, and the difficulties and distresses to which great numbers of Seamen, worn out and become decrepit in the King's service in consequence of the war, must unavoidably be exposed, unless some provision could be made for their support during the remainder of their lives, and the Court being of opinion that they had no authority from Parliament to appropriate any part of the revenue towards making provision for those who could not be accommodated within the Hospital; it was resolved unanimously to make immediate application to Parliament for leave to bring in a Bill to empower the Commissioners and Governors * (after defraying the necessary expences of the Hospital) to provide for such of the above-mentioned Seamen as could not be received into it; and a Bill for this purpose being presented by the late Mr. Grenville, re- 3 G. 3. ceived the Royal assent on the 31st of March, 1763.

* The funds of the Hospital are not applicable to the payment of Out-Pensioners, when the revenue is not more than sufficient for its proper establishment; and, in that case, Parliament has (on application) voted specific sums for that purpose.

them

In confequence of which 1400 Out-Penfioners were appointed at 7l. per Ann. each; whofe numbers gradually
decreafed in confequence of death, or admiffion into
the Hofpital, till the year 1782, when 500 additional
ones were appointed, and in the year following as
many more; the In-Penfioners who were defirous of
it, were allowed to retire upon the Out - Penfion,
if they thought proper and there appeared to be no
objection.

Perfons defirous of becoming Out-Penfioners, apply at the Admiralty Office in the fame manner as the
others above-mentioned, and, when appointed, take their
Warrants to the Treafurer's Office at the Hofpital, where
a ticket is delivered to them, by which they are empowered to receive their penfion by quarterly payments,
either at that place, or if, at a great diftance, from the
Collectors of the Cuftoms or Excife, in confequence of
Certificates figned and tranfmitted by the Treafurer, and
attefted by the Steward, or Clerk of the Checque.

About 2650 Out-Penfioners have been admitted from
the paffing of the above-mentioned Act to the prefent
time.

N. B. By the above - mentioned Act, " All affign-
" ments, bargains, fales, orders, contracts, agreements, or
" fecurities whatfoever, which fhall be given or made by
" any Out-Penfioner, for, upon, or in refpect of, any fum or
" fums of money, to become due on any Out-Penfion granted
                                                    " by

4

" *by the Commiffioners or Governors of the Hospital, fhall be ab-*
" *folutely null and void to all intents and purpofes.*"

Alfo, " *the perfonating or falfely affuming the name and*
" *character of an Out-Penfioner of Greenwich Hofpital in*
" *order to receive the Out-Penfion, or procuring any other to*
" *do the fame, is made felony without benefit of Clergy.*"

N   THE

PAINTED-HALL.

THE painting of this Hall, which is executed in a mafterly manner, was undertaken by Sir James Thornhill, in 1708.

In the cupola of the veftibule is reprefented a Compafs with it's proper points duly bearing. And in the covings, in chiaro ofcuro, the Four Winds with their different attributes.

Over each of the three doors are compartments, in chiaro ofcuro, (fupported by boys fuppofed to be the fons of poor Seamen) containing the names of the feveral Benefactors to the Hofpital; and above, in a niche, is the figure of Charity.

In this veftibule is the model of an antique Ship, prefented by the late Lord Anfon; the Original, which is of marble and was found in the Villa Mattea in the 16th centuary, now ftands before the Church-of Sta. Maria in Rome, hence called Sta. Maria in Navicella.

From this veftibule a large flight of fteps leads into the Saloon, or grand Hall, which is about 106 feet long, 56 wide, and 50 high; ornamented with a range of Corinthian

rinthian pilafters ftanding on a Bafement, and fupporting a rich Entablature above. Between them, on the South-fide, are the windows, two rows in height, the jambs of which are ornamented with rofes impanelled. On the North-fide are receffes anfwering to the windows, in which are painted, in chiaro ofcuro, the following allegorical figures, viz. *Hof-pitalitas, Magnanimitas, Liberalitas, Mifericordia, Generofitas, Bonitas, Benignitas, Humanitas.*

In the frize around the Hall is the following in-fcription:

Pietas augufta ut habitent fecure et publice alantur qui pub-licæ fecuritati invigilarunt regia Grenovoci Mariæ aufpiciis fublevandis nautis deftinata regnantibus Gulielmo & Maria MDCXCIV.

Over the great arch, at the weft end, are the Britifh Arms fupported by Mars and Minerva, which are very finely fculptured.

On the Cieling are the portraits of King William and Queen Mary, the Royal Founders, furrounded by the Cardinal Virtues, &c. and with the emblematical repre-fentation of the Four Seafons of the Year; this Cieling is very well defcribed by Sir Richard Steel in his Lover; of which the following is a Copy:

" In the middle of the Cieling is a very large Oval frame
" painted and carved in imitation of gold, with a great
" thicknefs rifing in the infide to throw up the figures to the

" greater height; the Oval is faftened to a great Suffite adorned
" with rofes in imitation of copper. The whole is fup-
" ported by eight gigantic figures of Slaves four on each fide,
" as though they were carved in ftone; between the figures,
" thrown in heaps into a covering are all manner of Maritime
" Trophies in Metzo-relievo; as Anchors, Cables, Rudders,
" Mafts, Sails, Blocks, Capitals, Sea-guns, Sea-carriages,
" Boats, Pinnaces, Oais, Stretchers, Colours, Enfigns, Pen-
" nants, Drums, Trumpets, Bombs, Mortars, Small-arms,
" Granades, Powder-barrels, Fire-arrows, Grapling-irons,
" Crofs-ftaves, Quadrants, Compaffes, &c. all in ftone-colours,
" to give the greater beauty to the reft of the cieling, which
" is more fignificant.

" About the Oval in the infide are placed the twelve figns
" of the Zodiac; the fix northern figns, as Aries, Taurus,
" Gemini, Cancer, Leo, Virgo, are placed on the north fide
" of the Oval; and the fix fouthern figns, as Libra, Scorpio,
" Sagittarius, Capricornus, Aquarius, Pifces, are to the fouth,
" with three of them in a groupe, which compofe one quarter
" of the year: the Signs have their attitudes,* and their drape-
" ries are varied and adapted to the feafons they poffefs, as

* _Aries_ is of a turbulent afpeƈt with little winds and rains hovering about
him, his drapery of a blewifh green, fhadowed with dark ruffet to denote the
changeablenefs of the weather. _April_, or _Taurus_, is more mild ; _May_, or _Ge-_
mini, in blue ; _June_, a calm red ; _July_, more reddifh, and as he leans upon
his Lyon veils a little from the Sun. _Virgo_ almoft naked, and flying from the
heat of the Sun ; _Libra_ in deep red ; _Scorpio_ veils himfelf from the fcorching
Sun in a flame colour mantle ; _Sagittarius_ in red, lefs hot; _December_ or _Capri-_
corn, blewifh ; _Aquarius_ in a waterifh green ; _Pifces_ in blue. Over _Aries_,
Taurus, _Gemini_ prefides _Flora_ ; over _Cancer_, _Leo_, _Virgo_ prefides _Ceres_ ; over
Libra, _Scorpio_, _Sagittarius_, _Bacchus_; and over _Capricorn_, _Aquarius_, _Pifces_,
Hyems hovering over a brazen pot of fire.

" the

" the cool, the blue, and the tender green to the Spring, the
" yellow to the Summer, and the red and flame colour to
" the Dog-days and Autumnal feafon, the white and cold to
" the Winter; likewife the fruits and the flowers of every
" feafon as they fucceed each other.

" In the middle of the oval are reprefented King William
" and Queen Mary fitting on a Throne under a great pavi-
" lion, or purple canopy, attended by the four cardinal virtues,
" as Prudence, Temperance, Fortitude, and Juftice.

" Over the Queen's head is Concord, with the Fafces,
" at her feet two doves, denoting mutual concord and inno-
" cent agreement, with Cupid holding the King's Sceptre
" while he is prefenting Peace with the Lamb and Olive
" Branch, and Liberty expreffed by the Athenian cap to Eu-
" rope, who laying her Crowns at his feet receives them
" with an air of repefct and gratitude. The King tramples
" Tyranny under his feet, which is expreft by a French per-
" fonage with his leaden Crown falling off, his chains, yoke
" and iron fword broken to pieces, Cardinal's cap, triple
" crowned mitres, &c. tumbling down. Juft beneath is
" Time bringing Truth to light, near which is a figure of
" Architecture holding a large drawing of part of the Hof-
" pital with the Cupola, and pointing up to the Royal Foun-
" ders, attended by the little Genii of her art. Beneath her
" is Wifdom and Heroic Virtue, reprefented by Pallas and
" Hercules, deftroying Ambition, Envy, Covetoufnefs, De-
" traction, Calumny, with other vices, which feem to fall to
" to the earth, the place of their more natural abode.

" Over

" Over the Royal pavilion is fhewn at a great height
" Apollo in his golden chariot, drawn by four white horfes
" attended by the Horæ, and morning dews falling before
" him, going his courfe through the twelve figns of the
" Zodiac ; and from him the whole plafond or cieling is en-
" lighthened.

" Each end of the Cieling is raifed in perfpective, with a
" balluftrade and cliptic arches, fupported by groupes of ftone
" figures, which form a gallery of the whole breadth of the
" Hall; in the middle of which gallery (as though on the
" flock) going into the upper Hall, is feen in perfpective the
" Tafferil of the Blenheim man of war, with all her galleries,
" port-holes open, &c. to one fide of which is a figure of Vic-
" tory flying with fpoils taken from the enemy, and putting
" them aboard the Englifh man of war. Before the fhip is
" a figure reprefenting the City of London, with the arms,
" fword and cap of maintenance, fupported by Thame and
" Ifis, with other fmall rivers offering up their treafures to
" her. The river Tine pouring forth facks of coals. In
" the gallery on each fide the fhip are the Arts and Sciences
" that relate to Navigation with the great Archimedes, many
" old philofophers confulting the compafs, &c.

" At the other end, as you return out of the Hall, is a
" gallery in the fame manner, in the middle of which is the
" ftern of a beautiful galley filled with Spanifh trophies.
" Under which is the Humber with his pigs of lead. The
" Severn with the Avon falling into her, with other leffer
" rivers. In the North end of the gallery is the famous Ticho
" Brahe, that noble Danifh Knight, and great ornament of
" his

" his profeſſion and human nature. Near him is Copernicus
" with his Pythagorean fyſtem in his hand; next to him is
" an old mathematician holding a large table, and on it are
" deſcribed two principal figures, of the incomparable Sir
" Iſaac Newton, on which many extraordinary things in that
" art are built.   On the other end of the gallery, to the ſouth,
" is our learned Mr. Flamſtead, Reg. Aſtron. Profeſſ. with
" his ingenious diſciple, Mr Thomas Weſton.   In Mr.
" Flamſtead's hand is a large ſcroll of paper, on which is
" drawn the great Eclipſe of the Sun that will happen in
" April————1715; near him is an old man with a pen-
" dulum counting the ſeconds of Time, as Mr. Flamſtead
" makes his obſervations with his great mural arch and
" tube on the deſcent of the moon on the Severn, which at
" certain times form ſuch a roll of the tides as the ſailors
" corruptly call the Higre, inſtead of the Eager, and is very
" dangerous to all ſhips in its way.   This is alſo expreſſed by
" rivers tumbling down by the moon's influence into the
" Severn.   In this gallery are more Arts and Sciences relating
" to Navigation.

    " All the great rivers, at each end of the Hall, have their
" proper product of fiſh iſſuing out of their vaſes.

    " In the four great angles of the Cieling, which are over
" the arches of the galleries, are the four elements, as Fire,
" Air, Earth, and Water, repreſented by Jupiter, Juno,
" Cybele, and Neptune, with their leſſer Deities accompa-
" nying, as Vulcan, Iris, the Fauni, Amphitrite, with all
" their proper attitudes, &c.

                                        " At

" At one end of the great Oval is a large figure of Fame
" defcending, riding on the winds, and founding forth the
" praifes of the Royal Pair.

" All the fides of the Hall are adorned with fluted Pi-
" lafters, Trophies of fhells, Corals, Pearls ; the jambs of the
" windows ornamented with rofes impanneled, or the opus
" reticulamium, heightened with green gold.

" The whole raifes in the fpectator the moft lively images
" of Glory and Victory, and cannot be beheld without much
" paffion and emotion."

From this Saloon you afcend, by another flight of fteps, into
the upper Hall, the Cieling and Sides of which are adorned
with different paintings. In the centre of the cieling is
reprefented Queen Ann and Prince George of Denmark
accompanied with various emblematical figures.

In the four corners are the Arms of England, Scotland,
France, and Ireland, between which are the four quarters
of the world, Europe, Afia, Africa and America, with the
emblems and productions of each.

On the left hand fide as you enter is a painting in imitation of Baffo Relievo reprefenting the landing of the Prince
of Orange, afterwards King William. On the right hand
over the chimney is the landing of King George the Firft at
Greenwich.

At the further end of this Hall are painted the portraits of King George the Firft and his Family, with
many emblematical figures ; amongft which the Painter
(Sir James Thornhill) has alfo introduced his own portrait.

On

On the right and left of the entrance are allegorical paintings reprefenting *The Public Weal*, and *Public Safety*.

The whole of this celebrated work was not completed till 1727, and coft 6,685*l.* being after the rate of 3*l.* per yard for the Ceiling and 1*l.* per yard for the Sides, agreeable to a refolution of the Directors, after confulting the following eminent Painters, viz. Vandervelt, Cooper, Richardfon, Sykes, and Degard, who reported the performance to be equal to any of the like kind in England, and fuperior in number of figures and ornaments.

When Sir James had finifhed the Ceiling and Sides of the great Saloon in 1717, he delivered in a Memorial to the Directors, ftating the prices which were given for paintings of the like kind at the Banqueting-Houfe, Whitehall, the Duke of Montague's, the Palaces of Windfor and Hampton-Court, Bulftrode-Chapel, and other works at the Duke of Portland's, and at the Earl of Burlington's, which is too curious to be omitted, and the following copy of it is therefore inferted :

To the Right Honourable the Commiffioners for building the Royal Hofpital at Greenwich.

The Memorial of James Thornhill, Hiftory-Painter,

Sheweth,

That, in purfuance of an order of the 10th Inft. fignified to me by Mr. Corbet that I fhould make a demand and valuation of the Painting done by me at the faid Hofpital, I have made diligent enquiry into the prices of Hiftory Painting in this kingdom, and find, that when

O money

money was at much greater value, greater prices were given, and beg leave to inftance in one, not prefuming to a parallel. Sir Peter Paul Rubens had 4,000*l.* for the ceiling of the Banqueting-Houfe, at Whitehall, which is little more than 400 yards of work, fo was near 10*l.* a yard..

The late Duke of Montague paid Mons.ʳ Roffo for his Salloon 2,000*l.* and kept an extraordinary table for him, his friends and fervants, for two years, whilft the work was doing, at an expence computed at 500*l. per Ann.;* which is near 450 yards, amounting to about 7*l.* per yard, ceiling and fides..

Sign.ʳ Varrio was paid for the whole Palaces of Windfor and Hampton Court, ceilings, fides, ftairs, and back-ftairs, 8*s.* per foot, which is 3*l.* 12*s.* per yard, exclufive of gilding, had wine daily allowed him, lodgings in the Palaces; and, when his eye-fight failed him, a penfion of 200*l. per Ann.* and allowance of wine for his life..

	£.
Sig.ʳ Rizzi had of the prefent Duke of Portland for 3 Rooms - - - -	1000
For the little Chapel at Bulftrode - - -	600
Of the Lord Burlington for his ftaircafe -	700
Sign.ʳ Pellegrini of the Duke of Portland for work at his houfe - - -	800
And for a fmall picture over a chimney -	50
Of the Earl of Burlington for the fides of his hall - - - - -	200

All

All which prices are by meafure, more than Sign*
Varrio's; and I was lately paid for a Ceiling at Hampton
Court, upon a reference from the Right Honourable the
Lords Commiffioners of his Majefty's Treafury to the
Honourable Board of Works, 3*l.* 15*s.* per yard, including
gilding. And, although thefe painters were foreigners, yet
fince the feveral ingenious Gentlemen painters and artifts,
to whom your Honours have been pleafed to refer this
for a parallel to be drawn, have not thought this inferior
in performance, and more full of work, I have no reafon
to apprehend any difcouragement from your Honours, but
that you will be pleafed to allow me as good a price as any
of thefe modern painters, efpecially fince I have fpent fix
years of the prime of my life therein; and, tho' I have in
that time done feveral fmall works, yet they have chiefly
ferved to enable me by experience and money to carry on
this great one, which muft otherwife neceffarily have required a confiderable impreft for which a large intereft
would have been paid.

And alfo hope that this being an Hofpital will make no
difference, fince Royal Hofpitals are as well embellifhed as
Palaces, and with as much experice. Therefore humbly
fubmit myfelf to your Honours juftice herein, and am,

Your Honours

Moft faithful, and

24th *Auguft,*
1717.

Obedient humble Servant,

JAMES THORNHILL.

O 2   CHAPEL.

C H A P E L.

THE interior part and roof of the former Chapel, which was executed under the direction of Mr. Ripley the Surveyor, being deftroyed by fire on the 2d of January, 1779, has been reftored in the moft beautiful and elegant ftyle of Grecian Architecture from defigns of the late Surveyor, James Stuart, Efq. the celebrated publifher of the Antiquities of Athens, and under the fuperintendance of Mr. William Newton, Clerk of the works.

Immediately before the Entrance of the Chapel is an Octangular veftibule in which are four niches containing the ftatues of Faith, Hope, Charity, and Meeknefs, worked from defigns made by Weft; from which veftibule you afcend, by a flight of 14 fteps, to the Chapel; which is 111 feet long and 52 broad, and capable of conveniently accommodating 1000 Penfioners, Nurfes, and Boys, exclufive of pews for the Directors, and for the feveral Officers, under officers, &c. Over the Portal or great Door of the Chapel is this infcription, in letters of gold:

" *Let them give thanks, whom the Lord hath redeemed, and delivered from the hand of the enemy.*" Pf. 107.

The portal confifts of an Architrave, Frize, and Cornice of ftatuary marble, the jambs of which are twelve feet high in one piece, and enriched with excellent fculpture. The

Frize

Frize is the work of Bacon, and confifts of the figures of two Angels with feftoons fupporting the facred Writings, in the leaves of which is the following infcription :

> " *The Law was given by* Mofes ;
> " *But Grace and Truth came by* JESUS CHRIST.

The great folding doors are of mahogany highly enriched, and the whole Compofition, of this Portal is not, at this time, to be paralleled in this, or, perhaps, in any other country.

Within this entrance is a Portico of fix fluted marble columns fifteen feet high. The capitals and bafes are Ionic, after Greek models. The Columns fupport the organ gallery, and are crowned with an entablature and balluftrade enriched with fuitable ornaments.

On the Tablet in the front of the gallery is a Baffo-relievo reprefenting the figures of Angels founding the Harp ; on the pedeftals, on each fide, are ornaments confifting of Trumpets and other inftruments of mufic ; and, on the tablet between, is the following infcription in letters of gold:

> "*Praife him with the found of the trumpet :*

> "*Praife him with ftringed inftruments and organs.*" Pf. 150.

I

In

In this gallery is a very fine Organ, made by Mr. Samuel Green.

On each fide of the Organ Gallery are four grand Columns; their fhafts of Scagliola in imitation of Sienna marble, by Richter, and their Capitals and Bafes of Statuary marble; At the oppofite end of the Chapel are four others of the fame fort, which fupport the arched Ceiling and Roof. Thefe Columns are of the Corinthian order, and, with their Pedeftals, are 28 feet high.

On the fides of the Chapel, between the upper and lower range of windows, are the two galleries, in which are pews for the Officers and their Families: thofe of the Governor and Lieutenant Governor, which are oppofite each other, are diftinguifhed by ornaments confifting of the Naval Crown, and other fuitable Infignia. Underneath thefe galleries, and the Cantilivers which fupport them, are ranges of fluted Pilafters. The Cantilivers are decorated with antique foliage; the Entablature over the Pilafters with Marine Ornaments; the interval between them with Feftoons, &c. and the Pedeftals of the Balluftrade in the front of the Galleries with Tridents and Wreaths. The tablets in the middle of each Balluftrade contain the Hofpital's arms, and the Frize below is carved with foliage in the Greek mode. Over the lower range of Windows are Paintings, in chiaro ofcuro, reprefenting fome of the principal events in the life of our Saviour, which are accompanied with ornaments of Candelabra and Feftoons.

Above

Above the Galleries is a richly-carved ftone Fafcia, on which ftands a range of Pilafters of the Compofite mode, their fhafts being of Scagliola, correfponding with thofe of the eight great columns, and, jointly with them, appearing to fupport the Epiftylium which furrounds the whole Chapel. This Epiftylium is enriched with Angels bearing feftoons of Oak-leaves, Dolphins, Shells, and other applicable ornaments. From this rifes the curved Ceiling which is divided into Compartments and enriched with foliage, golochi, &c. in the antique ftyle. Between the upper pilafters are recefles in which are painted, in chiaro-ofcuro, the Apoftles and Evangelifts.

At each end of the Galleries are concave recefles, the coves of which are ornamented with Coffers and Flowers carved in ftone ; in thefe recefles are the doors of entrance to the Galleries, decorated with enriched Pilafters and Entablatures, and a group of ornaments, confifting of the Naval Crown, wreaths of Laurel and Tridents. Above the doors are circular recefles, containing paintings, in chiaro-ofcuro, of the Prophets Ifaiah, Jeremiah, Mofes, and David.

The Communion Table is a femi-oval flab of ftatuary marble near eight feet long. The afcent to it is by three fteps of black marble, on which is fixed an ornamental railing reprefenting feftoons of Ears of Corn, and Vine foliage. This Table is fupported by fix Cherubin ftanding on a white marble ftep of the fame dimenfions.

4

Above is a Painting, by Weſt, in a ſuperb carved and gilt frame, repreſenting *the Preſervation of St. Paul from ſhipwreck on the Iſland of Melita.*

This picture is 25 feet high and 14 wide, and conſiſts of three principal groups. The firſt, which is at the lower part, repreſents the Mariners and Priſoners bringing on ſhore the various articles which have been preſerved from the wreck; Near theſe is an elegant figure, ſuppoſed to be a Roman Lady of diſtinction, claſping with affection an Urn containing the aſhes of her deceaſed huſband who had fallen in the wars of Judea. Before her is an aged, infirm Man; who, being unable to aſſiſt himſelf, is carried in the arms of two robuſt young men.

In the middle part of the piece is the principal group, confiſting of St. Paul ſhaking into the fire the Viper that had faſtened on his hand, the Brethren who accompanied him, his friend the Centurion, and a band of Roman Soldiers with their proper inſignia.

The figures above theſe, on the ſummit of the rocks, form the third group; and confiſt of the hoſpitable Iſlanders lowering down fuel and other neceſſaries for the relief of the Sufferers.

The Sea and wrecked Ship, (which at this point of time are conſidered as an epiſode) appear in the back-ground, and combine to exhibit a ſcene that cannot fail of having a proper effect on the minds of Sea-faring men, and of impreſſing them with a due ſenſe of their paſt preſervation,

vation, and their prefent comfortable fituation and fupport in this glorious Afylum for naval misfortune and
naval worth.

On either fide the arch which terminates the top of this
picture, are Angels of ftatuary marble as large as life, by
Bacon; one bearing the Crofs, the other the emblems of
the Eucharift. This excellent combination of the works
of art is terminated above in the fegment between the
great cornice and ceiling by a painting of the Afcenfion,
defigned by Weft, and executed by Rebecca, in chiaro
ofcuro; forming the laft of the feries of paintings of the life
of our Saviour which furround the Chapel.

The middle of the aile, and the fpace round the
altar and organ gallery, are paved with black and white
marble in golochi, frets, and other ornaments; having, in
the centre, an Anchor and Seaman's Compafs.

The Pulpit is on a circular plan, fupported by fix fluted
columns of Lime-tree, with an Entablature above richly
carved and of the fame material. In the fix Inter-columns
are the following alto-relievos, taken from the Acts of
the Apoftles, executed after defigns by Weft.

The Converfion of St. Paul,   Acts, chap. ix.
Cornelius's Vifion,   x.
Peter releafed from Prifon by the Angel,   xii.
Elymas ftruck blind,   xiii.
St. Paul preaching at Athens, and converting Dio-
     nyfius the Areopagite,   xvii.
Paul pleading before Felix,   xxiv.

P   The

The Reader's Defk is formed on a fquare plan, with columns at the four corners, and the Entablature over them fimilar to thofe of the Pulpit; in the four Inter-columns are alfo alto relievos of the Prophets, copied after defigns by the fame artift.

> Daniel.
> Micah.
> Zachariah.
> Malachi.

The following paintings, in chiaro-ofcuro relative to our Saviour, are placed over the lower windows.

The firft four of the feries, painted by De Bruyn, are at the Eaft end of the South-fide of the Chapel, and reprefent

> The Nativity.
> The Angel appearing to the Shepherds.
> The Magi worfhiping.
> The Flight into Egypt.

The four, which follow on the fame fide, are by Catton and reprefent

> St. John baptizing.
> Calling of St. Peter and St. Andrew,
> Our Saviour preaching from a Ship to the People on
>   Shore.
> The Stilling of the Tempeft.

The four, at the Weſt-end of the North-ſide, are by Milburne and repreſent

> Our Saviour walking on the Sea, and ſaving Peter
> from ſinking.
> The Blind Man cured by a Touch.
> Lazarus raiſed from the Dead.
> The Transfiguration.

The next four on the ſame ſide are by Rebecca and repreſent

> The Lord's Supper.
> Our Saviour carried before Pilate.
> The Crucifixion.
> The Reſurrection.

The Apoſtles and Evangeliſts in the receſſes between the upper windows, and the four Prophets in the circles above the Gallery-doors are by the laſt-mentioned Artiſt, after deſigns of Mr. Weſt.

The Principal Artificers who were employed in rebuilding the Chapel were:

> Mr. John Deval, Maſon.
> Mr. Richard Lawrence, Carver.
> Mr. Samuel Wyatt, Carpenter.
> Mr. James Arrow, Joiner.
> Mr. John Papworth, Plaiſterer.

P 2   COUNCIL-

N. B. The four ſtatues in the veſtibule of the Chapel—the medallions or alto-relievos in the Pulpit and Reading-deſk—the pannel of Cherubims with the Harp, and the two pannels of the Hoſpital Arms in front of the Galleries—the Cherubims ſupporting the Communion-table—all the Pilaſter Capitals, &c. are of artificial ſtone, executed at COADE's Ornamental Stone Manufactory, near Weſtminſter-bridge.

COUNCIL-ROOM.

ADJOINING to the Governor's Apartment in King Charles' Building is a Room fo called, where the Directors occafionally meet on the affairs of the Hofpital; and a Council is held every Friday, (or oftner if neceffary,) by the Officers intrufted with the internal Government of the Penfioners, &c.

In this Room are feveral paintings.

At the upper-end is a whole-length Portrait of King George the Second in his Robes, by Schakleton, the bequeft of a former Governor, Admiral Townfend.

On each fide of it are two half-lengths, one of K. William, the other of Queen Mary, by Sir Godfrey Kneller, the gift of the late Sir John Van Hattem, Knight, of Dinton Hall, Bucks.

At the lower-end is a whole-length Portrait, by Gainfborough, of the prefent Earl of Sandwich, the gift of Sir Hugh Pallifer, Bart. the prefent Governor.

On the right is a half-length Portrait, by Sir Peter Lely, of Edward the firft Earl of Sandwich, who was killed in the engagement in Solbay in 1672, the gift of the prefent Earl.

On the left is a half-length of Lord Vifcount Torrington, by Davifon.

Over

Over the Chimney is a whole-length Portrait of Robert
Ofbolfton, Efq. (whofe munificent benefaction has already
been noticed) copied from an original in the poffeffion of
Lord Aylmer, a former Governor, at the expence of the Hofpital, by Degard.

On the right hand of the chimney is a whole-length Portrait of Lord Vifcount Torrington, by Davifon, in 1734.

On the left a ditto, by Richardfon, of Admiral Sir John
Jennings, a former Governor.

Near the window at the upper end of the room is a three
quarters Oval of Captain Clements, a former Lieutenant Governor, by Greenhill, pupil of Sir Peter Lely, the gift of the
Captain's Widow.

At the lower-end the Head of a venerable old Man, faid
to have been the firft Penfioner who was admitted into the
Hofpital.

In the Pannel oppofite the Chimney is a Spring-Clock, by
Holmes, ornamented with the Signs of the Zodiac, beautifully
carved and gilt, from a defign of the late Mr. Stuart, when
Surveyor of the Hofpital.

Under feveral of the above Pictures are fome of Sir James
Thornhill's original fketches, for the Paintings in the Great
Hall, prefented by the faid Mr. Stuart, and Mr. Cox of Bad-
bey, Northamptonfhire.

A N T I-

ANTI-CHAMBER *to the* COUNCIL-ROOM.

Near the Door is a Month Equation Clock with a double Pendulum, by Quire; And, in different parts of the Room, the following Paintings, viz.

Two large Sea Pieces, given by Philip Harman, Efq; reprefenting the Naval exploits of his Anceftor, Captain Thomas Harman, in the Reign of King Charles II ; One, at the upper-end of the Room, being an engagement between the Tyger Frigate commanded by Captain Harman and eight Dutch Privateers, in oppofition to which he conducted a large Fleet of Colliers into the River Thames, without the lofs of one, when there was the greateft want of Coals in London ; The other, over the Door at the lower-end, being an engagement between the fame Captain, in the fame Frigate and a Dutch Man of War, in the Bay of Bulls; in which the latter was taken and towed into the Harbour of Cadiz, in fight of a Squadron of Dutch fhips riding there.

In other parts of the Room are fix fmall Pictures reprefenting the Lofs of the Luxemburgh Galley, commanded by William Kellaway (which was burnt in the year 1727, on her paffage from Jamaica to London) and the fubfequent diftreffes of part of her crew ; the gift of Mr. Parker, Executor to Captain Maplefden, late Lieutenant-Governor of the Hofpital. As the circumftances of this difafter are interefting and extraodinary, we are induced to give the following fhort account as related by Captain Boys himfelf, late Lieutenant-Governor of the Hofpital, who was fecond Mate of the fhip at that time.

"On

" On the 23d day of May, 1727, we failed from Ja-
" maica, and on Sunday the 25th day of June were in
" the latitude of 41°, 45′ N. and in the longitude of 20′,
" 30′ E. from Crooked Ifland, when the galley was per-
" ceived to be on fire in the Lazaretto.   It was occafioned
" by the fatal curiofity of two black boys, who, willing
" to know whether fome liquor fpilt on the deck was
" rum, or water, put the candle to it, which rofe into
" a flame, and immediately communicated itfelf to the
" barrel from whence the liquor had leaked.   It had
" burned fome time before it was perceived, as the boys
" were too much intimidated to difcover it themfelves.
" Having tried all poffible means to extinguifh the fire in
" vain, we hoifted out the yaul, which was foon filled
" with 23 men and boys, who had jumped into her with
" the greateft eagernefs.   The wind now blowing very
" frefh, and fhe running 7 knots and a half by the log,
" we expected every moment to perifh, as fhe was loaded
" within a ftreak and a half of her gunnel.   We had
" not a morfel of victuals, nor a drop of liquor ; no maft,
" no fail, no compafs to direct our courfe, and above a
" hundred leagues from any land.   We left 16 men in
" the fhip, who all perifhed in her : they endeavoured to
" hoift out the long-boat, but, before they could effect
" it, the flames reaching the powder-room, fhe blew up,
" and we faw her no more.   A little before this we could
" diftinguifh the Firft Mate, and the Captain's Cook
" in the mizen-top, every moment expecting the fate
" that awaited them.   Having thus been eye-witnefses
" of the miferable fate of our companions, we expected
" every moment to perifh by the waves, or, if not by

' them,

" them, by hunger and thirſt. On the two firſt days it
" blew and rained much, but the weather coming fair on
" the third day, viz. the 28th, as kind providence had
" hitherto wonderfully preſerved us, we began to contrive
" means how to make a ſail, which we did in the follow-
" ing manner: we took to pieces three mens' frocks and
" a ſhirt, and with a ſail-needle and twine, which we
"foun d in one of the black boy's pockets, we made ſhift
" to ſew them together, which anſwered tolerably well.
" Finding, in the ſea, a ſmall ſtick, we woulded it to a
" piece of a broken blade of an oar that we had in the
" boat, and made a yard of it, which we hoiſted on an
" oar with our garters for halyards and ſheets, &c. A
" thimble, which the fore-ſheet of the boat uſed to be
" reeved through, ſerved at the end of the oar or maſt to
" reeve the halyards. Knowing, from our obſervations, that
" Newfoundland bore about North, we ſteered as well
" as we could to the northward. We judged of our courſe,
" by taking notice of the Sun and of the time of the
" day by the Captain's watch. In the night, when we
" could ſee the North-ſtar, or any of the Great Bear, we
" formed the knowledge of our courſe by them. We
" were in great hopes of ſeeing ſome ſhip, or other, to
" take us up. The 4th or 5th night a man, Thomas
" Craniford, and the boy that unhappily ſet the ſhip on
" fire, died, and, in the afternoon the next day, three more
" men, all raving mad, crying out miſerably for water.
" The weather now proved ſo foggy, that it deprived us
" almoſt all day of the ſight of the Sun, and of the
" Moon and Stars by night. We uſed frequently to holloo
" as loud as we coud, in hopes of being heard by ſome
                                      " ſhip.

" fhip. In the day-time our deluded fancies often imagined
" fhips fo plain to us, that we have hollooed out to them
" a long time before we have been undeceived ; and, in the
" night, by the fame delufion we thought we heard men
" talk, bells ring, dogs bark, cocks crow, &c. and have
" condemned the phantoms of our imagination (believing
" all to be real fhips, men, &c.) for not anfwering and
" taking us up. The 7th day we were reduced to 12 in
" number, by death. The next night, the wind, being about
" E. N. E, blew very hard, and the fea running high,
" we fcudded right before it with our fmall fail about
" ¼ down, expecting every moment to be fwallowed up by
" the waves. July the 5th, Mr. Guifhnet died, and on
" the 6th died Mr. Steward, (fon of Dr. Steward, of Spa-
" nifh-Town, in Jamaica) and his fervant, both paffengers.
" In the afternoon we found a dead duck which looked
" green, and not fweet ; we eat it however very heartily,
" (not without thanks to the Almighty) and it is impoffible
" for any body, except in the like unhappy circumftances,
" to imagine how pleafant it was to our tafte at that time,
" which, at another, would have been offenfive both to our
" tafte and fmell. On the 7th day of July, at one in the after-
" noon, we faw land about fix leagues off. At 4 o'clock another
" man died, whom we threw overboard to lighten the
" boat. Our number was then reduced to feven. We
" had often taken thick fog banks for land, which as often
" had given us great joy and hopes that vanifhed with
" them at the fame time ; but when we really faw the land,
" it appeared fo different from what we had fo often taken
" for it, that we wondered how we could be fo miftaken,

Q   " and

" and 'tis abfolutely impoffible for any man, not in our circum-
" ftances, to form an idea of the joy and pleafure it gave us
" when we were convinced of its reality. It gave us ftrength
" to row, which we had not for four days before, and muft
" infallibly moft of us, if not all, have perifhed that very
" night, if we had not got on fhore. Our fouls exulted
" with joy and praifes to our Almighty Preferver. About
" 6 o'clock we faw feveral fhallops fifhing, which we
" fteered for. Having a fine gale of wind right on fhore,
" we went with fails and oars, about three or four knots :
" when we came fo near that we thought one of the
" fhallops could hear us (being juft under fail and going in
" with their fifh) we hollooed as loud as we could ; at length
" they heard us, and lowered their fail. When we ap-
" proached pretty near them, they hoifted it in again, and
" were going away from us ; but we made fo difmal and
" melancholy a noife, that they brought to and took us in
" tow. They told us our afpects were fo dreadful, that
" they were frightened at us. They gave us fome bread
" and water ; we chewed the bread fmall with our teeth,
" and then by mixing water with it, got it down with
" difficulty.

" During our voyage in the boat, our mouths had been
" fo dry for want of moifture for feveral days, that we
" were obliged to wafh them with falt water every two
" or three hours to prevent our lips glewing faft together.
" We always drank our own water, and all the people
" drank falt water, except the Captain, Surgeon, and my-
" felf. In foggy weather the fail having imbibed fome
" moifture, we ufed to wring it into a pewter bafon which

" we

" we found in the boat.   Having wrung it as dry as we
" could, we fucked it all over, and ufed to lick one another's
" clothes with our tongues.   At length we were obliged
" by inexpreffible hunger and thirft to eat part of the
" bodies of fix men, and drink the blood of four ; for we
" had not fince we came from the fhip faved, only one
" time, about half a pint, and, at another, about a wine
" glafs full of water, each man in our hats.   A little food
" fufficing us, and finding the flefh very difagreeable, we
" confined ourfelves to the hearts only.   Finding ourfelves
" now perifhing with thirft, we were reduced to the me-
" lancholy, diftrefsful, horrid act of cutting the throats of
" our Companions, an hour, or two, after they were dead,
" to procure their blood, which we caught in a pewter
" bafon, each man producing about a quart.   But let it
" be remembered in our defence, that without the affift-
" ance this blood afforded to nature, it was not poffible
" that we could have furvived to this time.   At about
" 8 o'clock at night we got on fhore at Old St. Lawrence
" Harbour in Newfoundland, where we were kindly re-
" ceived by Captain Lecrafs of Guernfey, or Jerfey,
" then Admiral of the Harbour.   We were cautioned to
" eat and drink but little at firft, which we obferved as
" well as the infirmity of human nature, fo nearly ftarving,
" would allow.   We could fleep but little, the tranfports
" of our joy being too great to admit of it.   Our Captain,
" who had been fpeechlefs 36 hours, died about 5 o'clock
" the next morning, and was buried with all the Honors
" that could be conferred upon him at that place.   The
" names of thofe perfons who were burnt in the fhip,
" who were ftarved in the boat, and who lived to get on
" fhore, are as follow, viz.

Q 2

" Ralph

Burnt in the Ship.

Ralph Kellaway, 1st Mate.
Isaae Holroide, 3d Mate.
Jerald Hedge, Gunner..
James Crook, Cooper..
John Johnson,
William Coats,
William D..y,   } Seamen.
James Ambrose,

Charles James,
Francis Mitto,   } Seamen..
Tho* Hino,. Quarter Master..
Edward Thicker,
Evander Mc Avy, } Seamen..
Sharper,
Jemmy,   } Black Boys..
Coffea,.

Starved in the Boat..

Thomas Steward, Paffenger..
Mr. Stewards, Servant.
William Piggs, Paffenger..
John Horn,
John Eaft,
Henry White,   } Seamen..
Tho* Croniford,
Simon Emar,

William Walker,
John Simenton,
William James,   } Seamen..
Tho* Nicholfon,
Henry Guifhnett, Clerk..
Caufor,.
Hamofe,   } Black Boys..
Merry Winkle,

Lived to get on Shore.

William Kellaway, Captain.   William Gibbs, Carpenter..
William Boys, 2d Mate..   Robert Kellaway, a Boy.
Thomas Scrimfour, Surgeon..   George Mould,. Seaman..
William Batten, Boatfwain..

"The boat in which we got to Newfoundland, diftance
"100 leagues, was only 16 feet long, 5 feet 3 inches broad,
"and two feet 3 inches deep.. It was built for the Lux-
"burgh Galley, by Mr. Bradley, of Deal."

N. B. Lieut. Governor Boys was accuftomed to pafs annually in prayer and fafting the number of days the fhip's
crew were in diftrefs as above-mentioned; in commemo-
ration of his wonderful deliverance.

INFIRMARY.

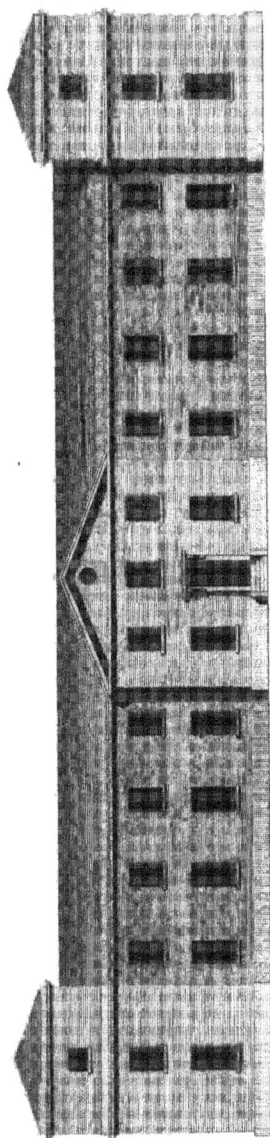

INFIRMARY.

IN 1763 it was submitted to the General Court by the Directors whether it would not be adviseable to build an Infirmary without the Walls of the Hospital; in order that more Penfioners might be added to the establishment, and the fick taken care of with greater convenience and more comfort to themfelves.

A work fo neceffary was immediately concluded upon, and a Building ordered to be erected for that purpofe; which was defigned by Mr. Stuart the late Surveyor, and completed under the direction of Mr. Robinfon then Clerk of the Works.

It is a quadrangular brick Building 198 feet in length, and 175 feet in breadth; and divided into two principal parts, one for the Patients under the care of the Phyfician, and the other for thofe whofe Cafes require the attendance of a Surgeon.

Each part is two ftories in height, containing a double row of rooms being altogether in number 64, calculated to hold 256 Patients; each room has a Chimney-place, with an aperture near the Ceiling for the purpofe of ventilation, and will accommodate four Patients.

In

In the fore-part of this Building, which confifts of the Phyfician's divifion, is the Hall ; oppofite to it, in the back part which belongs to the Surgeon, is the Kitchen ; and, in the upper ftory, is a fmall Chapel, where prayers are read by the Chaplains, twice a week, for the benefit of the Patients.

In the four angles and other parts of the building, are the Difpenfary and Surgery and apartments for the Phyfician ; for the Surgeon and Difpenfer, with their refpective Affiftants ; and for the Matron ; and adjacent, within the walls, are hot and cold Baths.

As nothing has been omitted which was judged necef-fary to render this building convenient and comfortable to the Patients, fo all poffible care is taken that the Diet (a fcheme of which is annexed) is adapted to their parti-cular Cafes ; the Drugs and Medicines are bought of the Apothecaries Company in order that they may be the beft of their kinds; and, when it is neceffary for any of the Patients to go to Bath, or the falt-water, or, in Cafes of Infanity, to Bethlem or other places of confine-ment, they are immediately fent thither; the Hofpital paying all neceffary expences.

TABLE

TABLE of DIET.

Days.	Bread. lb.	Beer. Quarts	Veal. lb.	Muttⁿ lb.	Beef. lb.	Milk. Quarts	Butter lb.	Eggs. No.	Sugar. lb.	Rice. lb.
Sunday	1	1	$\frac{1}{4}$	—	—	—	—	---	---	---
Monday	1	1	—	—	—	1	$\frac{1}{6}$	2	$\frac{1}{6}$	---
Tuesday	1	1	—	$\frac{1}{4}$	—	—	—	---	---	---
Wednesd.	1	1	—	—	—	—	$\frac{1}{6}$	2	$\frac{1}{6}$	---
Thursday	1	1	—	—	$\frac{3}{4}$	—	—	---	---	---
Friday	1	1	—	—	—	1	$\frac{1}{6}$	2	$\frac{1}{6}$	$\frac{1}{4}$
Saturday	1	1	—	$\frac{1}{4}$	—	—	---	---	---	---
Total per Week	7	7	$\frac{1}{4}$	$1\frac{1}{2}$	$\frac{1}{4}$	2	$\frac{1}{2}$	6	$\frac{1}{2}$	$\frac{1}{4}$

N. B. Water-gruel for breakfaſt and milk-pottage for ſupper on meat days; panada for breakfaſt and rice-milk for ſupper on banyan days. Wine, aſſes milk, &c. are ſupplied according to the demands of the Phyſician and Surgeon.

By

The following T A B L E fhews the Number of Penfioners who died in the laft twelve Years.

	Jan.	Feb.	Mar.	April	May	June	July	Aug.	Sept.	Oct.	Nov.	Dec.	Total.
1777	18	13	15	13	11	18	11	15	19	16	21	15	185
1778	18	11	11	22	16	19	11	19	16	16	21	14	194
1779	19	18	25	22	16	13	16	15	19	19	15	18	215
1780	30	19	17	21	15	17	15	13	17	25	15	20	224
1781	14	15	16	18	22	11	15	18	16	23	15	23	206
1782	16	19	15	21	24	31	18	16	16	16	17	19	228
1783	18	15	17	14	12	17	13	15	16	17	15	19	188
1784	17	25	21	25	22	14	13	6	6	10	10	17	186
1785	20	16	14	16	14	18	21	19	15	15	10	17	195
1786	11	20	20	12	13	20	8	18	15	7	24	8	176
1787	36	14	12	20	11	16	14	11	14	16	27	21	212
1788	13	15	22	20	13	11	16	15	15	14	12	25	191
Total	230	200	205	224	189	205	171	180	184	194	202	216	-----2400

N. B. By this Table it appears that a number exceed-
ing the whole of the prefent complement, viz. 2350, has
been buried in the above-mentioned period.

SCHOOL.

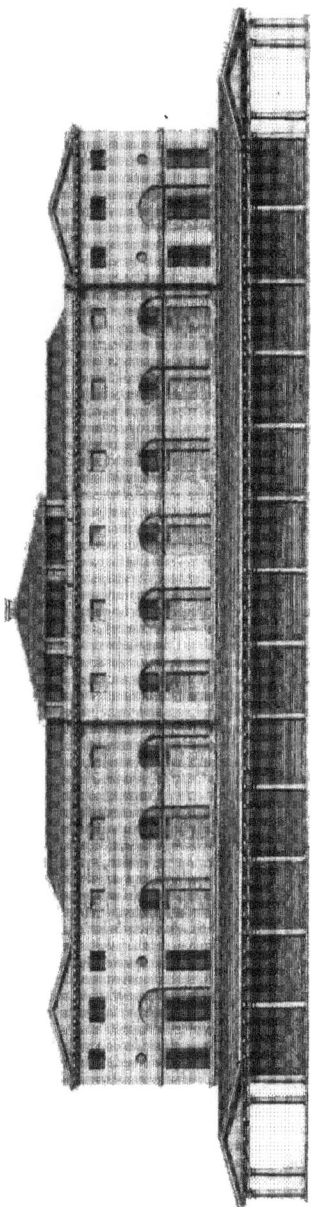

S C H O O L.

AGREEABLE to the tenor of King William's Commiffion, and the Regifter Act, which direct fome Provifion to be made for the Maintenance and Education of the Sons of Seamen, it was ordered by the Governor and Council, in the year 1715, that 10 Boys fhould be inftructed in Reading, Writing, and Navigation, by Mr. Wefton, Mathematical Mafter in the Town of Greenwich; and put out Apprentices to Mafters of fhips or others.

In 1719, Rules were fettled by the Directors, and afterwards confirmed by a General Court, for the admiffion, maintenance, and education of Seamens Sons.

In 1731, their number amounted to 60 and has from time to time been further augmented to 150, (the prefent complement) as the increafing ftate of the funds appropriated for them has admitted of it.

This Eftablifhment is folely under the management of the Directors, who in rotation nominate the boys for admiffion; prior to which it muft be made appear, by proper Certificates, that they are

Sons of Seamen.
Between eleven and thirteen years of age.
Objects of Charity.
Of found body and mind, and able to read.

R   And

And their Parents or Friends muſt give ſecurity that they
ſhall be at the Directors diſpoſal, and to indemnify the
Hoſpital for the value of their clothes &c. if they ſhould
run away with them.

The Boys are lodged, clothed, and maintained, at the expence of the Hoſpital, for three years.

Five Nurſes are appointed to keep them clean, to take
care of their clothes, to make their beds, attend at their
meals, &c. And a Guardian and four Aſſiſtants, are appointed to ſuperintend them when out of School.

They are inſtructed in the principles of Religion by the
Chaplains, and in Writing, Arithmetic and Navigation by
a School Maſter appointed for that purpoſe; who alſo in-
ſtructs thoſe in Drawing who ſhew a genius for it.

Each Boy, on his admiſſion, is ſupplied with a Bible and
Common Prayer Book, and with all neceſſary Books and In-
ſtruments for his inſtruction, which he is allowed to take
with him when he is bound out.

All the Boys attend the Directors, once a year to be
viewed; when they bring ſpecimens of their ſeveral perfor-
mances; and three of them who produce the beſt Drawings
after nature, done by themſelves, are allowed the following premiums, according to their reſpective degrees of
merit, viz.

                                        A Hadley's.

A Hadley's Quadrant, 1ft Prize.
A Cafe of Mathematical Inftruments, 2d Ditto.
Robertfon's Treatife on Navigation, 3d Ditto.

They are bound out for feven years, to the fea-fervice only, for the better improvement of their talents, and that they may become able Seamen and good Artifts.

In 1783, it was recommended by the Directors to the General Court, to build a School, and Dormitory, for the Boys, without the walls of the Hofpital, that they might be better accommodated, and the rooms which they occupied in the Hofpital converted to Wards for the reception of more Penfioners, whenever it might be found neceffary to take in an additional number.

Accordingly a Building, defigned by Mr. Stuart, the late Surveyor, was erected near the Hofpital, under the fuper-intendance of Mr. Newton, Clerk of the Works.

This Building is 146 feet in length, and 42 in breadth, exclufive of its Tufcan Colonade intended for a play-place and fhelter for the boys in bad weather, which is 180 feet long, and 20 feet broad.

In this Building is a School-Room 100 feet long, and 25 broad, capable of containing 200 Boys; in the two ftories above are Dormitories of the fame fize, fitted up with Hammocks for the Boys to fleep in. Adjoining are Rooms for

R 2

the

the Guardian, Nurfes, and other neceffary attendants;
and, at a fmall diftance, a good Houfe for the Schoolmafter.

This excellent Charity, which is calculated for the double
purpofe of providing for the fons of poor Seamen and making them ufeful to their country, by training them up to a
Seafaring life, has been, and is folely fupported by money
arifing from the following incidental funds, viz.

Shewing the Painted Hall, Chapel, and other parts of the
Hofpital.

Mulcts, abfences, Cheques, &c. of Penfioners, and
Nurfes.

Profits on Provifions purchafed of the Penfioners. *

Sale of old Houfhold ftores.

Unclaimed property of deceafed Penfioners and Nurfes.

Intereft of Money in the Stocks, being favings from the
above-mentioned funds.

The Clothing of the Boys, as well Linen as Woollen, is of
the fame quality as that of the Penfioners, and they are new-
clothed as often as the Directors think fit ; and when bound
out, are fupplied with two complete fuits, and other
neceffaries.

* By this excellent plan, thofe who find it more convenient for their familes
to have money in lieu of their provifions, are prevented from expofing them
to fale elfewhere ; and though the Hofpital derives a profit, are allowed full
as much if not more than they can otherwife make of them.

They

They eat altogether at a Table provided for them within
the Hofpital; and the following is a fcheme of their diet
for every day in the week, viz.

Days.	Bread. oz.	Beer. Quarts	Beef. lb.	Muttⁿ lb.	Rice Milk. Pint.	Plumb Puddᵇ lb.	Peafe Soup. Pint.	Butter oz.	Cheefe oz.
Sunday	14	1	—	¼	—	—	—	—	2
Monday	14	1	—	—	1	—	—	1	2
Tuefday	14	1	—	¼	—	—	—	—	2
Wednefd.	14	1	—	—	—	¼	—	1	2
Thurfday	14	1	½	—	—	—	—	—	2
Friday	14	1	—	—	—	—	1	1	2
Saturday	14	1	—	¼	—	—	—	—	2
Total per Week.	98	7	½	1¼	1	¼	1	2	14

Broth is allowed on each Meat day.

About 2,650 Boys have been admitted from the firſt
Eſtabliſhment to the prefent time.

After

After the foregoing account of the present state of the spot whereon several of our former Monarchs have resided, it may not be unacceptable to our Readers to see a Description and View of the old Palace, which, by the Favour of the Antiquarian Society, we are enabled to annex.

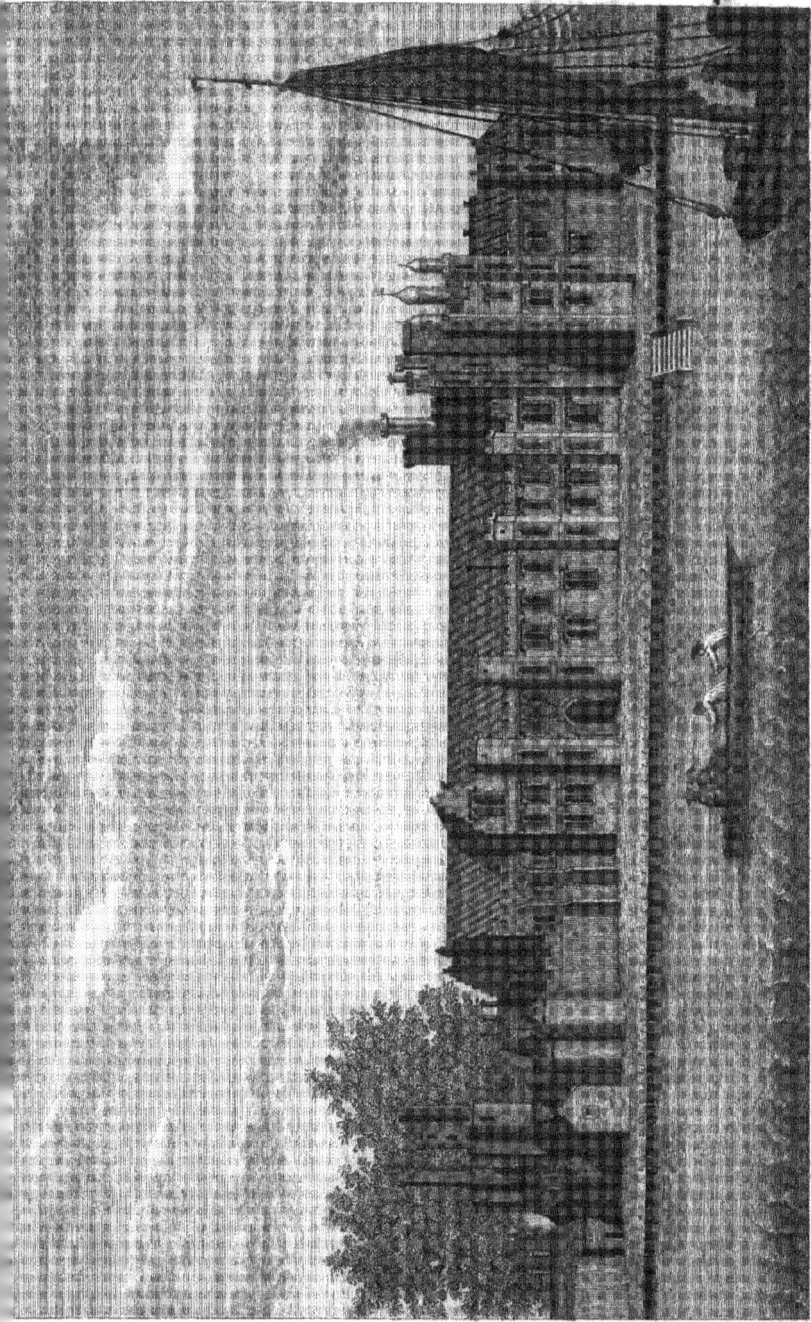

A View of the ANCIENT ROYAL PALACE, call'd, PLACENTIA, in East Greenwich.

Copied from an Engraving published by the Society of Antiquaries of London.

Published Sept.r 22, 1794 by the Rev.d John Nichols and John Nichols, F.A.S.

Engraved by Newton.

AN ACCOUNT OF THE

Ancient ROYAL PALACE of PLACENTIA,

IN

E A S T - G R E E N W I C H.

GREENWICH, or Grenewick, *vicus viridans*, called, in ancient Deeds and other Writings, Eaft - Grenwick, in order to diftinguifh it from Deptford, which was heretofore called. Weft-Greenwick, probably from its Situation on the verdant Banks of the Thames.

Before we mention the Palace, it may not be improper to give fome Account of the Lands on which it was erected. They, together with Lewifham, Woolwich, and other Appendages, were given to the Church of St. Peter, in Ghent, by Elftrude, Niece to King Edgar, and Wife to Baldwin, Earl of Flanders, for the Health of her Soul, and the Souls of her Hufband and his two Sons, Arnulf and Adenulf.

Dunftan, Archbifhop of Canterbury, who had been Abbot of St. Peter's, at Ghent, is faid to have prevailed upon King Edgar to renew and confirm the aforefaid Grant by his Charter, dated 964. The fame Grant was renewed by Edward the Confeffor, William the Conqueror, Henry I, II, and King John. Pope Eugenius and his Succeffor Alexander,

ander confirmed thefe Royal Grants ; but a Difpute arifing between the Abbot and Convent of Ghent, and the Bifhop of Rochefter, concerning the Churches of Eaft Greenwich and Lewifham, the fame Claim was by Pope Clement referred to Baldwin, Archbifhop of Canterbury, whereupon thofe Churches were appropriated to the Abbey of Ghent, Anno 1218, which Sentence was confirmed by Richard, Bifhop of Rochefter, Anno 1239.

By Domefday Book it appears, that, foon after the Conqueft, the Manor of Greenwich, as Parcel of the Poffeffions of the Bifhop of Lifieux, paid Service to Odo, Bifhop of Bayeux, and Earl of Kent.

King Edward I, by Letters Patent, bearing Date at Weftminfter, the 5th of May, Anno Regni 3°, granted a Licence to the Abbot and Convent of St. Peter's at Ghent, to fell the faid Manors of Lewifham and Greenwich, with their Apurtenances, to Walter, Bifhop of Rochefter, to be held by him and his Succeffors of the King of England, and his Heirs in *capite*.

The Alien Priories being, by Parliament, given to King Henry V, in the Second Year of his Reign [a], this Prince, the Year after, granted the Manors of Lewifham and Greenwich, &c. formerly belonging to the Abbey of St. Peters at Ghent, to his new erected Carthufian Abbey of Sheene.

[a] Rot. Parl. a° 2do Hen. V. n. 19.

The

The Palace, of which a View is engraven, from a Drawing in the Poffeffion of Dr. Ducarel, was begun by Humphrey, Duke of Gloucefter, in the Reign of Henry VI, who alfo granted his Royal Licence to the Duke and Alienora his Wife, to inclofe the Park, and afterwards to build a Tower or Caftle, which was finifhed by Henry the Seventh. The Duke is faid to have given the Name of Placentia to this Palace and Diftrict, on Account of their agreeable Situations; but Stow afferts that this Name was given by Henry the Seventh. King Edward IV, enlarged the Edifice; and in the 5th Year of his Reign, granted it to Elizabeth, his then Queen[b]. Henry VII, added a Brick Front towards the Water-fide, and built a Houfe adjoining to the Palace, probably the low Building, which is at the Eaft End thereof for the Reception of certain Obfervant Fryers, who came to Greenwich about the latter End of the Reign of K. Edward the Fourth, from whom they had obtained a Chauntry there, together with a fmall Chapel of the Holy Crofs. This Houfe, together with the Manors of Lewifham and Eaft Greenwich, being con-veyed, and affured, to King Henry VIII, his Heirs, and Succeffors, in the Twenty-fecond Year of his Reign[c]; he fpared no Coft to render it a fplendid and magnificent Pa-lace. Queen Elizabeth made feveral Additions to thefe Buildings; another Front towards the Gardens was built by Queen Ann, Wife of K. James I, who alfo laid the Foundation of the Houfe, next the Park, where the Go-vernor of the Hofpital afterwards refided, which Houfe was

[b] Pat. 5 Edw IV. p. 1. m. 15.   [c] Rot. Clauf. 22 Hen. VIII. m. 13.

S finifhed

finifhed and adorned in a fuperb Manner by Henrietta Maria, Queen to King Charles the Firft.

In this fair Palace, in which the Kings and Queens of England heretofore have taken fo great a Delight, were born many Royal Perfons; amongft others, Henry VIII, and his brother Edmund, and Edw. VI, Queen Mary, and her Sifter Queen Elizabeth, and feveral Children of K. James I. Here alfo died that moft amiable and ever lamented Sovereign Edward VI.

Henry Howard, Earl of Northampton, founded an Hofpital here, by the Thames, and enlarged and beautified the Edifice, which was then called the Caftle, being a more eminent Part of the King's Old Palace; from whence was a moft delightful Profpect towards the River.

An Ordinance[d] of Parliament paffed July 16, 1649, for the Sale of the Crown Lands, in which was a Claufe, providing, that the fame fhould not extend, *inter alia*, to the Manor of Eaft Greenwich, nor to the Houfe, Park, Caftle, or any Buildings thereunto belonging : in Confequence whereof they were permitted to remain in the Hands of the State.

The Neceffities of the Commonwealth, fome time after, requiring Monies to be raifed for defraying the Expences of the Navy; the Houfe of Commons, on the 27th of November, 1652, took that Matter into Confideration,

[d] Scobel's Acts,

and.

and came to the following Resolution; viz. That Greenwich House, Park, and Lands, should be immediately sold
for ready Money[e]. On the sixth of December[f] following
they ordered Surveyors to be sworn for the due Valuation of
the Premisses, in like manner as had been prescribed for
surveying other Estates of the late King, Queen, and Prince;
and on the 31st Day of the same Month, the House passed
an Ordinance for carrying the Survey and Sale into Execution. The Survey was accordingly taken, and Particulars
made out for the Sale of the Hoby Stables, and some
trifling Parts of the Royal Garden and Palace[g], but no
further Proceedings appear to have been had at that
Time.

In the Year 1654, the[h] Sub-Committee, for the Revenue,
finding that the House and Park of East Greenwich, together, with Hampton-Court House and Park, Somerset
House, &c. and other the King's Palaces, had been sur-
veyed, and the Buildings valued at 25,969l. 6s. 6d. but that
the same then remained unsold, after solemn Debates, declared, as their Opinion, that they are fit Places for the
Accommodation of the Lord Protector, therefore not to be
valued at any gross Sum, yet, that they might be allowed
toward the Revenue as they are returned in the Survey, at
the Rent of 1254l. 13s. 4d.

[e] Journals of the House of Commons, Vol. VII. p. 222.
[f] Ibid.
[g] Records in the Augmentation Office.
[h] Report of the Sub-Committee of Parliament for the Revenue, Anno 1654.
MS. in the Possession of Lord Godolphin.

King Charles the Second, finding the Old Palace greatly decayed by Time, and the Want of neceffary Reparations during the Ufurpation, foon after his Return to England, began to erect a New Palace in this Place ; but it being left unfinifhed at his Death, remained in that Condition until King William III. and Queen Mary, by Letters Patent, bearing Date the 25th of October, in the Sixth Year of their Reign, granted to Sir John Sommers, then Keeper of the Great Seal, and divers others, a Piece or Parcel of Ground, Part of the Manor of Greenwich, containing Eight Acres, Two Roods, and Thirty-two fquare Perches, and which, as defcribed in thofe Letters Patent, is bounded by the River Thames on the North, and contained, by Admeafurement, along the River, from a Houfe in the Occupation of Nicholas Smythys, to the Eaft End of the Edifice called the Veftry, Six Hundred Seventy-three Feet, abutting in Part, Eaft, on the public Way, leading from the Crane to the Back Lane, South on the Old Tilt-Yard and the Queen's Garden, and Weft on the Fryer's Road and other Lands belonging to the Crown, together with the Capital Meffuage, then lately in building by King Charles the Second, and ftill remaining unfinifhed, commonly called by the Name of the Palace at Greenwich, and there ftanding upon Part of the aforefaid Ground : To hold, forever, as of the Manor of Eaft Greenwich, in free and common Socage, by Fealty only, to the Intent that the Premiffes fhould be converted (as they have accordingly been) into an Hofpital for Seamen.

A LIST

A LIST of the present DIRECTORS *of the*
HOSPITAL.

Sir Hugh Pallifer, Bart.
James Fergufon, Efq.
Sir Alexander Hood, K. B.
Right Honourable William Eden.
Timothy Brett, Efq.
John Clevland, Efq.
John Tauzia Savary, Efq.
George Marfh, Efq.
William Wells, Efq.
Reverend John Cooke.
John Campbell, Efq.
Joah Bates, Efq.
Sir Richard Bickerton, Bart.
William Allen, Efq.
Martin Fonnereau, Efq.
Jofiah Hardy, Efq.
William Palmer, Efq.
William Thornton Aftell, Efq.
George Rogers, Efq.
Richard Hulfe, Efq.
Chriftopher Mafon, Efq.
Richard Prefton, Efq.
John Yenn, Efq.
William Bellingham, Efq.

A LIST

A LIST *of the* Lords High Admirals, *and* First Lords of the Admiralty, *and also of the* Masters *and* Governors, Lieutenant-Governors, Captains, Lieutenants, *and other Civil and Military Officers of the* Hospital, *from the Institution to the present Time.*

LORDS HIGH ADMIRALS and FIRST LORDS of the ADMIRALTY.

In 1694, Edward Ruffel, Esq;
1697, Edward Ruffel, Earl of Orford
1699, John Egerton, Earl of Bridgwater
1701, Thomas Herbert, Earl of Pembroke
1702, His Royal Highnefs Prince George of Denmark, Lord High Admiral
1708, Thomas Earl of Pembroke and Montgomery, Lord High Admiral
1709, Edward Ruffel, Earl of Orford
1710, Sir John Leake, Knt.
1712, Thomas Wentworth, Earl of Stafford
1714, Edward Ruffel, Earl of Orford
1717, James Berkeley, Earl of Berkeley
1727, George Byng, Vifcount Torrington
1733, Sir Charles Wager, Knt.
1742, Daniel Earl of Winchelfea and Nottingham
1744, John Duke of Bedford
1748, John Montagu, Earl of Sandwich
1751, George Lord Anfon
1756, Richard Earl Temple
1757, Daniel Earl of Winchelfea and Nottingham

1757, George

LORDS HIGH ADMIRALS.

In 1757, George Lord Anſon
    1762, George Montagu Dunk, Earl of Halifax
    ——, Right Hon. George Grenville
    1763, John Montagu, Earl of Sandwich
    ——, John Percival, Earl of Egmont
    1766, Sir Charles Saunders, K. B.
    ——, Sir Edward Hawke, K. B.
    1771, John Montagu, Earl of Sandwich.
    1782, Auguſtus Viſcount Keppel
    1783, Richard Viſcount Howe
    ——, Auguſtus Viſcount Keppel
    ——, Richard Viſcount Howe
    1788, John Pitt, Earl of Chatham.

MASTERS and GOVERNORS.

In 1708, Sir William Gifford, Knt.
    1714, Mathew Aylmer, Eſq.
    1720, Sir John Jennings, Knt.
    1744, Sir John Balchen, Knt.
    1746, Right Hon. Lord Archibald Hamilton
    1754, Iſaac Townſend, Eſq.
    1765, Sir George Bridges Rodney, Bart.
    1771, Francis Holbourn, Eſq.
    ——, Sir Charles Hardy, Knt.
    1780, Sir Hugh Palliſer, Bart.

LIEU-

LIEUTENANT-GOVERNORS.

In 1704, Captain John Clements
1705, ———— Robert Robinfon
1718, ———— Thomas Cleafby
——, ———— Jofeph Soanes,
1737, ———— Teudor Trevor
1740, ———— Charles Smith
1750, ———— Francis Danfays
1754, ———— James Lloyd
1761, ———— William Boys
1774, ———— Thomas Baillie
1778, ———— Jarvis Maplefden
1781, ———— Broderick Hartwell
1784, ———— James Fergufon

C A P T A I N S.

In 1704, Robert Robinfon
1705, Benjamin Hofkins
1712, Thomas Monk
1714, Thomas Cleafby
1717, Edmund Clark
1718, Thomas Smith
——, John Smith
1722, William Paulkner
1725, Charles Chamberlain
1728, Baron Wylde
——, Charles Smith

1736, Teudor

In 1736, Teudor Trevor
    1737, Robert Mann
    1740, Edward Gregory
    1743, Thomas Lawrence
    1745, Francis Danfays
    1747, James Lloyd
    1750, Peter Ofborne
    1753, Cotton Dent
    1754, James Rycaut
   ——, Juftinian Nutt
    1758, Elliot Smith
    1759, Richard Clements
    1761, Thomas Baillie
    1767, James Hobbs
    1769, Henry Marfh
    1770, Jarvis Maplefden
    1772, Thomas Allwright
    1774, Francis Lynn
    1775, James Cook
    1776, James Chads
    1779, George Robinfon Walters
    1781, John Gore

LIEUTENANTS.

In 1704, Pierce Welch
  ——, John Conftable
    1705, Edward Smith
    1709, Thomas Grimftone

T

1724, Henry

In 1724, Henry Power
1728, John Lambert
1736, William Carr
1739, Alexander Barclay
1743, Ifaac Power
1745, Henry Ofborn
1747, John Bray
1748, Alexander Gordon
-----, Henry Moyle
1749, Charles Stuterville
1750,, George Grant
1754,. James Cummings
1759, Charles Beffon
1766, Robert Kerr
-----, William Lefebvre
1772, Jofeph Neville
1773, Henry Smith
1774,. William Anfel
1778, Anthony Fortye-
1780, George Spearing
1782, William Lurcock
1783, Henry Mafters
1786, William Hunter
1787, Patrick Stuart

TREASURERS.

In 1695, John Evelyn
1704, William Draper
17⁺⁺, Galfredus Walpole
1721, Philip Cavendiſh
1736, Hercules Baker
1745, James Gunman
1754, Charles Saunders
1766, Alexander Hood

SECRETARIES.

In 1695, William Vanburgh
1716, Thomas Corbett
1736, William Corbett
1751, John Corbett
1753, Daines Barrington
1756, Philip Stephens
1759, John Milnes
1762, John Ibbetſon

AUDITORS.

In 1707, Sidney Godolphin
1733, James Hunter
1741, Charles Clarke

T 2   1742, Heneage

In 1742, Heneage Legge
1747, Swinfen Jervis
1757, Richard Huffey
1770, Edward Thurlow
1771, William Eden

C H A P L A I N S.

In 1705, Philip Stubbs
-----, Robert Barry
1716, Thomas Pocock
1738, Nicolas Tindal
1745, David Campbell
1772, John Cooke
1773, John Maule

P H Y S I C I A N S.

In 1704, Salifbury Cade,
1713, William Maundy
1714, William Oliver
1716, Richard Morton
1730, Peter Jouneau
-----, Stephen Hall
1731, David Cockburn
1762, Montague Bacon
1766, James Hoffack

S T E W-

STEWARDS.

In 1704, Jofeph Gafcoigne
   1717, William Bell
   1761, John Ellis
   1772, John Izard
   1774, John Godby

SURGEONS.

In 1704, James Chriftie
   1714, Ifaac Rider
   1754, Charles Allen
   1763, Henry Tom
   1764, John Holden
   1765, Benjamin Denham
   1766, William Taylor

CLERKS of the CHEQUE.

In 1718, Edward Smith
   1736, John Maule
   1776, Stephen John Maule

DISPENSERS.

In 17$\frac{12}{}$, Henry Blakey
   1757, John Pocock

SUR-

S U R V E Y O R S.

In 1696, Sir Chriſtopher Wren, Knt.
    1716, Sir John Vanbrugh, Knt.
    1726, Colin Campbell
    1729, Thomas Ripley
    1758, James Stuart
    1788, Sir Robert Taylor, Knt.
    ———, John Yenn

C L E R K S of W O R K S.

In 1696, John Scarborough
    ———, Henry Symmons
    1698, Nicholas Hawkeſmore
    1705, John James
    1746, William Robinſon
    1775, Robert Mylne
    1782, William Newton

T H E   E N D.

ERRATA.
Page 101, line 18, for *between,* read *beneath.*
In the Liſt of Directors, for *Richard,* read *Robert Preſton,* Eſq.